PROGRESS IN CLINICAL AND BIOLOGICAL RESEARCH

RECENT TITLES

Please contact the publisher for information about previous titles in this series.

The Use of Transrectal Ultrasound in the Diagnosis and Management of Prostate Cancer

THE USE OF TRANSRECTAL ULTRASOUND IN THE DIAGNOSIS AND MANAGEMENT OF PROSTATE CANCER

Proceedings of a Meeting held in Detroit,
Michigan, September 11–12, 1986

Editors

Fred Lee
Richard D. McLeary
St. Joseph Mercy Hospital
McAuley Health Center
Ann Arbor, Michigan

ALAN R. LISS, INC. • NEW YORK

Address all Inquiries to the Publisher
Alan R. Liss, Inc., 41 East 11th Street, New York, NY 10003

Copyright © 1987 Alan R. Liss, Inc.

Printed in the United States of America

Library of Congress Cataloging-in-Publication Data

The Use of transrectal ultrasound in the diagnosis and
    management of prostate cancer.

    (Progress in clinical and biological research ;
v. 237)
    Includes index.
    1. Prostate gland—Cancer—Diagnosis—Congresses.
2. Diagnosis, Ultrasonic—Congresses. I. Lee, Fred,
1930—   . II. Series. [DNLM: 1. Prostatic Neoplasms—diagnosis—congresses. 2. Prostatic Neoplasms—
therapy—Congresses. 3. Ultrasonic Diagnosis—
congresses.   WI PR668E v.237 / WJ 752 U84 1986]
RC280.P7U84   1987   616.99'463   87-4181
ISBN 0-8451-5087-1

Contents

viii / Contents

Contributors

H. Bertermann, Department of Urology, Christian-Albrechts-University, Kiel, Germany **[177]**

Simon Carter, Academic Unit, Institute of Urology, University of London, London, England **[xi]**

K.T. Evans, Academic Department of Radiology, University Hospital of Wales, Cardiff, U.K. **[161]**

Albert Goldstein, Departments of Ob/Gyn and Radiology, Wayne State University, Detroit, MI 48201 **[31]**

Jerry M. Gray, Department of Pathology, St. Joseph Mercy Hospital, Ann Arbor, MI 48106 **[15]**

G.J. Griffiths, Department of Radiology, Gwent Urological Centre, St. Woolos Hospital, Newport NPT 4SZ, U.K.**[161]**

H.H. Holm, Department of Ultrasound, Herlev Hospital, Herlev, Denmark **[143]**

Robert P. Huben, Department of Urologic Oncology, Roswell Park Memorial Institute, Buffalo, NY 14263 **[153]**

D.R. Jones, Academic Department of Radiology, University Hospital of Wales, Cardiff, U.K. **[161]**

Glen H. Kumasaka, Department of Radiology, St. Joseph Mercy Hospital, Ann Arbor, MI 48106 **[57]**

Fred Lee, Department of Radiology, St. Joseph Mercy Hospital, Ann Arbor, MI 48106 **[73]**

Peter J. Littrup, Department of Radiology, St. Joseph Mercy Hospital, Ann Arbor, MI 48106 **[143, 213]**

Richard D. McLeary, Department of Radiology, St. Joseph Mercy Hospital, Ann Arbor, MI 48106 **[49, 209]**

Gerald P. Murphy, School of Medicine, State University of New York at Buffalo, Buffalo, NY 14214 **[1, 219]**

W.B. Peeling, Department of Urology, Gwent Urological Centre, St. Woolos Hospital, Newport NPT 4SZ, U.K.**[161]**

Paul Ray, Division of Urology, Cook County Hospital and the University of Illinois College of Medicine, Chicago, IL 60612 **[111]**

E.E. Roberts, Academic Department of Radiology, University Hospital of Wales, Cardiff, U.K. **[161]**

P.G. Ryan, Department of Urology, Gwent Urological Centre, St. Woolos Hospital, Newport NPT 4SZ,U.K. **[161]**

Manfred H. Soiderer, Department of Pathology, St. Joseph Mercy Hospital, Ann Arbor, MI 48106 **[125]**

Soren Torp-Pedersen, Department of Ultrasound, Herlev Hospital, Herlev, Denmark **[143]**

Hiroki Watanabe, Department of Urology, Kyoto Prefectural University of Medicine, Kyoto, Japan 602 **[5,133,195]**

The numbers in brackets are the opening page numbers of the contributors' articles.

Preface

This symposium was the first of what is hoped to be an annual event, and reflected the rapidly growing interest in prostatic ultrasound in the United States. The meeting was run along the same lines as one of Dr. Lee's teaching sessions at Ann Arbor with additional contributions from many international authorities.

The well known conundrum of a high incidence of tumours of the prostate in post mortem studies as opposed to the clinical incidence was discussed in relation to diagnosis by ultrasound. There are 79 deaths/100,000 males in the USA from prostatic carcinoma, but the incidence of latent carcinoma in cadavers is approximately 30% of males over the age of 50, thus for every person dying of the disease, there are 380 people with prostatic carcinoma alive and well. The progression to clinical disease is not relentless and the selection of patients at risk is required. The preliminary results of ultrasound screening were reported as only detecting an incidence of 3%. Tumours as small as 3mm. in diameter have been detected by ultrasound using the new techniques and equipment; it is difficult to understand why the detection rate remains so small.

The importance of the size of the primary tumour in relation to the prognosis was described and this opens an exciting area for transrectal ultrasound. It was shown that tumours of less than 1.0 cc are extremely unlikely to metastasize and are of consistently better histological differentiation. The volumetric assessment of tumours by ultrasound is thus a useful prognostic indicator.

Lectures on how to perform a transrectal ultrasound examination of the prostate for detection of carcinoma gave many useful points on technique and interpretation.

The importance of both axial and sagittal scanning was emphasized, being comparable to the extra information given by looking at a lateral film of the chest beside the P.A. film. The importance of using the correct transducer frequency to obtain an optimum focal zone was stressed and above all, it is this information that has changed the face of prostatic ultrasound in the last two years. A brilliant double act by Dr. Lee (radiologist) and Dr. Gray (pathologist) demonstrated the remarkable correlation between histopathological and ultrasound studies. A new staging classification by ultrasound criteria was suggested but it remains to be seen whether this will be widely adopted, as the subtle demarcations proposed may be too complex and liable to mis-interpretation.

Certain themes emerged from this conference. The spectacular evaluation of ultrasound scans by whole prostate histology convinced everyone that the diagnostic criteria for early carcinoma have completely changed in the last two years. However, it is now realised that all tumours are neither all black or white, nor indeed all in the posterior zone. The importance of sagittal scanning for the accurate localisation of malignant lesions was evident. The diagnosis must always be substantiated by biopsy, best performed by obtaining both a tissue core and simultaneous aspiration specimens for cytology. The role of transcrectal ultrasound of the prostate has been extended into screening, staging and therapy. New developments in technology can be expected to increases still further the use of transrectal ultrasound in the management of prostatic carcinoma.

Simon Carter
London, England

The Use of Transrectal Ultrasound in the Diagnosis and
Management of Prostate Cancer, pages 1–3
© 1987 Alan R. Liss, Inc.

PROSTATE CANCER 1986:
WHERE HAVE WE BEEN AND WHERE ARE WE GOING?

Gerald P. Murphy, M.D., D.Sc.

School of Medicine, State University of New York
at Buffalo, 139 Parker Hall, Buffalo, New York
14214

Regardless of whether one uses the American classification or the TNM system of prostate cancer tumor staging,
the major concern of clinicians has been that of clinical
evaluation of prostatic cancer either on a preoperative
basis or for other decisions on therapy. This concern, of
course, remains unsettled and to some degree uncertain.
This grade and stage of the tumor are for example insepar-
ably related (Murphy, 1980) (Murphy, 1981 - Cancer).
Although this does not generally contribute to individual
decisions for specific patients, these are still important
factors when considering response to therapy in groups of
patients. With regard to the matter of histological grading
with whatever system is employed, the primary tumor of more
patients has been graded in the past years as documented by
the recent report of the American College of Surgeons
Commission on Cancer (Schmidt, 1986). Independently with
grade, survival characteristics are also currently available and most important (Schmidt, 1986).

Concerns over lymph node status based on operative
staging have been more recently limited to clinical trials
and less frequently in the general community used for
specific purpose (Murphy, 1980) (Murphy, 1981 - Cancer).
Lymph node transcutaneous fine needle aspiration is done by
some using lymphangiography with needle aspiration (Wajsman,
1982). CAT scanning has been used to a very limited degree.
All of these staging tests are recognized as having limited
accuracy in terms of false negative or false positive
results. The degree with which all appropriate pelvic
lymph nodes are necessarily fully visualized is a recognized

limitation. The problem of the ability of these tests to
detect microembolic and micrometastatic dissemination in
lymph nodes or elsewhere is unanswered, at least concept-
ually and for all practical purposes. Thus, for the present,
with regard to the past especially for these tests the
matter of the clinical or other staging of prostate cancer
has been mostly to determine whether the disease is confined
to the pelvis or whether it is disseminated based on lymph
node evaluation and bone scans and bone x-rays to detect
distal metastases (Murphy, 1981 - Ca) (Murphy, 1981 - Urol.).
Little really has recently changed without the use of transrectal ultrasonography in terms of pre-operative staging
and this, of course, will be the focus of this symposium.
We cannot otherwise suspect intraprostatic cancer that is
not palpable unless the specimen is removed.

However, this conference can and will evaluate the
applications of prostate visualization and staging with
ultrasonography. Ultrasonography cannot evaluate lymph
nodes. Ultrasonography (Pontes, 1984) has advanced the
clinical staging pre-operatively and indeed indirectly
therapeutically for localized prostate cancer, specifically
as a means of further refinement and detection of whether
or not the prostatic capsule has been violated grossly or
whether there is a likely extension into the seminal vesicles
(Pontes, 1984) (Lee, 1986). What has been most recently
defined to a different degree is that decreased echogenecity
has definitely been by consensus and experience at a few
centers identified to be associated and highly likely to
reflect prostatic cancer (Lee, 1986). That Lee and associates (1986) detected lesions at 1.5 centimeters or larger
may indirectly lead to further trials and further demon-
strations of earlier detection of prostate cancer and therefore hopefully to increasing the likelihood for cure. This
symposium will also contribute individual series and other
observations which will be published. More specifically,
improvements in technology both in terms of the actual
tumor aspiration or biopsy, as well as visualization and
other dimensions may readily be achieved (Boyce, 1986). As
Dr. Boyce has pointed out, using conventional transrectal
ultrasonography the biopsy rate is improved to about 86%
or better (Boyce, 1986). One can only expect this to improve
as mentioned with axialtomography with combinations of both
transrectal axial and hopefully with the introduction of
new equipment.

One can only say that prostatic ultrasonography has been a most productive area in cancer which has largely been advanced by individuals working in institutions throughout the world without grant support from our Federal Government. Industry has been a great support to the development of this, both in the United States and elsewhere. One can only hope for further advances.

REFERENCES

Boyce WH (1986). Editorial: Ultrasonography "Little Sir Echo,--". The Bulletin of the American Urological Association, Inc. 13(3):3-4.

Lee F, Gray JM, McLeary RD, Lee F Jr., McHugh TA, Solomon, MH, Kumasaka GH, Straub WH, Borlaza GS, and Murphy GP (1986). Prostatic Evaluation by Transrectal Sonography: Criteria for Diagnosis of Early Carcinoma. Radiology 158(1):91-95.

Murphy GP, Gaeta JF, Pickren J, and Wajsman Z (1980). Current Status of Classification and Staging of Prostate Cancer. Cancer 45(8):1889-1895.

Murphy GP (1981). The Diagnosis and Detection of Urogenital Cancers. Cancer 47(5):1193-1199.

Murphy GP (1981). Prostate Cancer: Continuing Progress. American Cancer Society, Inc. (Reprinted from Ca-A Cancer Journal for Clinicians Vol. 31 No. 2).

Murphy GP (1981). Prostate Cancer Today. Supplement to Urology 17(3):1-3.

Pontes JE, Ohe H, Watanabe H, and Murphy GP (1984). Transrectal Ultrasonography of the Prostate. Cancer 53(6): 1369-1372.

Schmidt JD, Mettlin CJ, Natarajan N, Pearce BB, Beart RW Jr., Winchester DP, and Murphy GP (1986). Trends in Patterns of Care for Prostatic Cancer, 1974-1983: Results of Surveys by the American College of Surgeons. J Urol 136: 416-421.

Wajsman Z, Gamarra M, Park JJ, Beckley SA, Pontes JE, and Murphy GP (1982). Fine-Needle Aspiration of Metastatic Lesions and Regional Lymph Nodes in Genitourinary Cancer. Urology 19(4):356-360.

The Use of Transrectal Ultrasound in the Diagnosis and
Management of Prostate Cancer, pages 5–13
© 1987 Alan R. Liss, Inc.

HISTORICAL PERSPECTIVES ON THE USE OF TRANSRECTAL
SONOGRAPHY OF THE PROSTATE

Hiroki Watanabe

Department of Urology, Kyoto Prefectural
University of Medicine
Kawaramachi-Hirokoji, Kyoto, Japan 602

EARLY ATTEMPTS

It may be a surprising fact that the history
of prostatic ultrasound started with an attempt at
transrectal sonography (TRS), which is currently
recognized as the most suitable procedure for the
purpose. The history of TRS is much longer than
that of contact compound scanning, which has become distributed so widely throughout the world.

On August 27, 1955, 31 years ago, Wild & Reid
presented their screw-type transrectal scanner
before the 4th Annual Conference on Ultrasonic
Therapy, held here, in Detroit, Michigan[1]. It is
a marvelous coincidence that we are now having
the first international symposium for TRS in the
same place where they reported the first work on
the method.

They constructed an intrarectal transducer
which was attached by cable to equipment which
gradually withdrew the transducer and rotated it
simultaneously. This was planned primarily for
diagnosing not the prostate but the rectum and
lower bowel.

The principle of their attempt was identical
with that of modern TRS, although they obtained
only a square-shaped picture presumably thought to
be a part of the rectal mucosa, because of the

poor state of electronic technology at that time.

By the way, I had been wondering for many years why their section of the rectum was square. When I first met with Dr. Wild later, I asked him the question directly. His answer was very simple. The display unit they used did not have a function to delineate a round shape.

Several urologists followed up on Wild's idea. Takahashi & Ouchi[3] reported on an A-mode presentation of the prostate via the transrectal route in 1963. Pell[4] and Gotoh & Nishi[5] independently published reports of similar methods in 1964 and 1965.

The A-mode presentation, however, could not reveal the distribution of the tissues in various phases. A more complete tomographic presentation was therefore required.

In 1964, Takahashi & Ouchi[6] developed a transrectal probe for radial scanning and obtained the first horizontal tomograms of the bladder and prostate. The poor quality of these early pictures, however, prevented them from having useful clinical application.

TRANSRECTAL SONOGRAPHY IN PRACTICAL USE

In the early autumn of 1967, just after finishing the Postgraduate Doctor Course in Tohoku University, Sendai, I was looking for some new diagnostic modality for the prostate. The idea I had first was an electric stethoscope to listen to the sound of the urinary stream in the urethra from the rectal cavity. Seeking for advice, I visited a cardiologist, Dr. Motonao Tanaka, chief of the medical electronics department in Tohoku University.

In his laboratory, I found a strange device. It was a special ultrasonic probe consisting of a steel pipe 50cm in length and 1cm in diameter with an oscillating disc at its tip. It had been newly developed by him to obtain the section of the heart via the esophagus. Currently cardiac sonography is easily available from the chest surface but at that time it was a big problem how to minimize the attenuation of ultrasound from air in the lung. Dr. Tanaka planned the new device to resolve the problem but was unable to use it on human subjects because its insertion into the esophagus caused too much pain. He was looking for another use for the device. Incidentally and luckily, I became involved in the situation. My poor idea for an intrarectal stethoscope was abandonned and we agreed enthusiastically to turn the device to get a prostatic section via the rectum.

The very next day, I took a patient with benign prostatic hypertrophy to Dr. Tanaka's laboratory. After much entreating and some threats he was laid on the bed and the probe inserted into his rectum. The section of the prostate we obtained was fantastic. It looked to me as if it was rose coloured[7,8].

From that time I began my daily pilgrimages to Dr. Tanaka's laboratory with patients suffering from various kinds of prostatic diseases to make TRS. But, strangely enough, the device never gave us again such fine tomograms as we had obtained in the first case. Afterwards the cause of the trouble was clarified as water leakage into the damper of the oscillating disc. However, if the tomogram had been too poor in that first case, I am not sure whether I would have become so much concerned with TRS. The impression from the first tomogram was so intense that I was convinced that good tomograms could be obtained when the attendant problems could be satisfactorily resolved. The goddess of fortune smiled only once on me.

In our early studies we placed the patient in the lithotomy position. In an attempt to improve the picture quality, we focused attention on the improvement of resolution and display characteristics.

As a result of these improvements, a tomogram was obtained which could be used for diagnostic application. But one problem remained with air bubbles seeping into the rubber balloon around the probe and often interfering with the transmission of the ultrasound. It took approximately one hour to remove the air bubbles on some occasions.

One day while in an art museum, I saw a modern sculpture ⋅ entitled "Magician's Chair" by a young Japanese artist. It was a fancy chair with a little wooden protrusion on the seat. This gave me the idea that the patient could be examined in the sitting position.

A prototype model of the equipment was constructed using this idea in 1972. With the balloon and the probe in the vertical position, the air bubbles would rise to the top of the balloon and not cause interference with the passage of the ultrasound. Moreover, the organs in the pelvic cavity, including the prostate and the bladder, were settled down to the bottom of the pelvis by gravity in this position, providing a very stable situation for examination.

After careful evaluation of the data obtained with this prototype model, we developed a more refined piece of equipment in 1973[9]. The equipment was streamlined yet again for commercialization in 1975[10][11].

Our first scanner for use in the lithotomy position had a function to show a longitudinal section with linear scanning by pulling down the inner tube manually. Saggital sections of the prostate using this function were published in 1970[2]. After careful evaluation, however, the function was omitted from the new equipment because the diagnostic capability in sagittal sections was thought to be less effective than that in horizontal sections.

After the completion of the special equipment for TRS, we sought to apply the method on a clinical basis. The size and volume measurement of the prostate by TRS was published in 1971[13][14] and the staging of prostatic cancer and the monotoring of treatment were mentioned in our paper in 1975[10].

By November, 1984, the number of patients submitting to examination in our clinic in Kyoto had reached 10,000. The rate of unsuccessful examination was only 0.6% and mostly from human factors[15].

The first publication of prostatic sonography in the U.S., using our former scanner for the lithotomy position, appeared in 1973 by King and associates[16]. This work was followed by Resnick and expanded as in now well known. He developed an original TRS scanner later in 1978[7]. The first publication in Europe with the same scanner was done in 1976 by Hallemans & Denis[8].

In 1980, Harada and associates[9], who were my former colleagues, originated the gray scale TRS. We also developed a pistol-type handy transrectal scanner in 1980[20].

In accord with the remarkable advancement of real-time ultrasound, a transrectal electronic linear scanner was realized and details were first published by Oka and associates[21] in 1982. This provides a longitudinal section which yields a real-time observation of urine flow through the urethra.

Lee and associates used this scanner for the detection of a small cancer focus inside the prostate in 1984. Recently they began to employ radial scanning too[22].

Saitoh and Watanabe[23][24] developed independently a special unit for interventional ultrasound, consisting of a transrectal electronic linear scanner and an attachment for needle guidance, for the puncture of the prostate and the seminal vesicles in 1981.

OTHER MODALITIES FOR PROSTATIC ULTRASOUND

Contact compound scanning was used very widely throughout the world in the 1970s as the standard procedure for general diagnostic ultrasound.
We tried this scanning to visualize the prostate
from the perineum in 1972 . Sections were obtain-
able but the quality of the picture was much worse
than that obtained by TRS. For that reason we
gave up this procedure.

Miller & Garvie reported on prostatic ultrasound from the abdominal surface by contact compound scanning in 1973. Some reports regarding
the same route using ordinary real-time scanner
are occasionally seen even now. However, TRS
gives far more information than abdominal ultrasound.

Transurethral A-mode ultrasound was first
done by Nishi in 1968. A tomographic representation via the transurethral route was reported by
Holm and associates   in 1974. Nakamura and
Niijima   designed independently a new transurethral probe unit and obtained a satisfactory tomogram of the bladder wall in 1978. Gammelgarrd &
Holm published a new probe for both transurethral
and transrectal use in 1980.

The prostate can also be delineated by transurethral scanning. However, information obtained
by this method is not basically different from
that obtained by TRS. Pain and the special skill
required for transurethral scanning may prevent
the method from being used routinely for the prostate.

REFERENCES

1) Wild JJ, Reid JM (1955). Echographic tissue
   diagnosis. Proc 4th Annual Conference on
   Ultrasonic Therapy: 1-26.
2) Wild JJ, Reid JM (1957). Progress in techniques of soft tissue examination by 15 MC pulsed
   ultrasound. In Kelly E (ed): "Ultrasound in

Biology and Medicine" Washington DC: American
Institute of Biological Sciences, pp30-45.
3) Takahashi H, Ouchi T (1963). The ultrasonic
diagnosis in the field of urology (The 1st report). Proc Jap Soc Ultrasonics Med 3: 7.
4) Pell RL (1964). Ultrasound for routine clinical investigations. Ultrasonics 2: 87-89.
5) Gotoh K, Nishi M (1965). Ultrasonic diagnosis
of prostatic cancer. Acta Urol Jap 11: 87-90.
6) Takahashi H, Ouchi T (1964). The ultrasonic
diagnosis in the field of urology (The 2nd report). Proc Jap Soc Ultrasonics Med 4: 35-37.
7) Watanabe H, Katoh H, Katoh T, et al (1968).
Diagnostic application of the ultrasonotomography for the prostate. Jap J Urol 59: 273-
279.
8) Watanabe H, Kaiho H, Tanaka M, et al (1971).
Diagnostic application of ultrasonotomography
to the prostate. Invest Urol 8: 548-559.
9) Watanabe H, Igari D, Tanahashi Y, et al (1974).
Development and application of new equipment
for transrectal ultrasonography. J Clin Ultrasound 2: 91-98.
10) Watanabe H, Igari D, Tanahashi Y, et al (1975).
Transrectal ultrasonotomography of the prostate. J Urol 114: 734-739.
11) Watanabe H (1979). Prostatic Ultrasound. In
Rosenfield AT (ed): "Genitourinary Ultrasonography" New York: Churchill Livingstone, pp
125-137.
12) Watanabe H, Kaiho H, Tanaka M, Terasawa Y
(1970). Ultrasonotomography of the prostate
(Second report)---Sagittal tomography of the
prostate using B-scope scanning. Proc Jap Soc
Ultrasonics Med 18: 37-38.
13) Kaiho H, Watanabe H, Tanaka M, Terasawa Y
(1971). Ultrasonotomography of the prostate
(Fourth report)---A measurement of the size of
the prostate. Proc Jap Soc Ultrasonics Med 20:
93-94.
14) Watanabe H, Igari D, Tanahashi Y, et al (1974).
Measurements of size and weight of prostate by
means of transrectal ultrasonotomography.
Tohoku J Exp Med 114: 277-285.
15) Watanabe H, Ohe H, Saitoh M, et al (1985). A
survey on 10,000 examinations by transrectal

ultrasonotomography in our clinic. Proc Jap
Soc Ultrasonics Med 47: 921-922.
16) King WW, Wilkiemeyer RM, Boyce WH, et al(1973).
Current status of prostatic echography. JAMA
226: 444-447.
17) Resnick MI, Boyce WH (1979). Ultrasonography
of the urinary bladder, seminal vesicles and
prostate. In Resnick MI, Sanders RC (ed)
"Ultrasound in Urology" Baltimore: Williams &
Wilkins, pp220-250.
18) Hallemans E, Declercq G, Denis L (1977). Transrectal ultrasonotomography. Eur Urol 3: 37-40.
19) Harada K, Tanahashi Y, Igari D, et al (1980).
Clinical evaluation of inside echo patterns in
gray scale prostatic echography. J Urol 124:
216-220.
20) Itakura Y, Ohe H, Saitoh M, Date S (1980).
Application of a handy-type transrectal scanner. Proc Jap Soc Ultrasonics Med 36: 365-
366.
21) Sekine H, Oka K, Takehara Y (1982). Transrectal longitudinal ultrasonotomography of the
prostate by electronic linear scanning.
J Urol 127: 62-65.
22) Lee F, Gray J, McLeary R, et al (1986). Prostate cancer---Diagnosis by transrectal ultrasound: New ultrasound criteria with histopathologic correlations. J Urol 135 (4, Part
2): p.147A.
23) Saitoh M, Watanabe H, Ohe H (1981). Ultrasonically guided puncture for the prostate and
seminal vesicles with transrectal real-time
linear scanner. J Kyoto Pref Univ Med 90:
47-53.
24) Abe M, Hashimoto T, Matsuda T, et al (1986).
Prostatic biopsy guided by transrectal ultrasonography using a real-time linear scanner.
Urology 28 (in print).
25) Watanabe H, Kaiho H, Shima M, et al (1972).
Ultrasonotomography of the prostate (6th report)---Transperineal contact scanning. Proc
Jap Soc Ultrasonics Med 21: 61-62.
26) Miller SS, Garvie WHH, Christie AD (1973).
The evaluation of prostate size by ultrasonic
scanning: A preliminary report. Brit J Urol
45: 187-191.

27) Nishi M (1968). Diagnosis of prostatic disease by application of ultrasonic A-scope indication. Act Urol Jap 14: 3-40.
28) Holm HH, Northeved A (1974). A transurethral ultrasonic scanner. J Urol 111: 238-241.
29) Nakamura S, Niijima T (1980). Staging of bladder cancer by ultrasonography: A new technique by transurethral intravesical scanning. J Urol 124: 341-344.
30) Gammelgaard J, Holm HH (1980). Transurethral and transrectal ultrasonic scanning in urology. J Urol 124: 863-868.

The Use of Transrectal Ultrasound in the Diagnosis and
Management of Prostate Cancer, pages 15–29
© 1987 Alan R. Liss, Inc.

Prostate Gland: Anatomy, Hyperplasia, Cytologic Atypia,
Adenocarcinoma, and Tumor Markers.

Jerry M. Gray, M.D.

Department of Pathology, St. Joseph Mercy Hospital, Ann Arbor, Michigan 48106

ANATOMY

The structure of the prostate gland is complex and it
changes during maturation and aging. There is disagreement
as to the subdivisions of the prostate gland into various
lobes (Tisell et al, 1984). However, the descriptions of
McNeal which include a peripheral zone, central zone, and
anterior fibromuscular area (McNeal, 1984) have practical
clinical value in terms of the kinds of diseases which tend
to develop in the peripheral zone (carcinoma, cytologic
atypia) as compared with the central zone and the anterior
fibromuscular region (benign hyperplasia).

BENIGN HYPERPLASIA

Normal prostate glands weigh 20 gm plus or minus 6 in
men between the ages of 21 and 30 and this weight remains
constant with increasing age unless benign prostatic hyperplasia (BPH) develops (Berry et al, 1984). The frequency of
hyperplasia is only 8% at fourth decade; however, 50% of men
have pathologic BPH when they are 51 to 60 years old. The
average weight of a prostate that is recognized at autopsy
to contain benign hyperplasia is 31 gm plus or minus 16.
Only 4% of the prostates in men more than 70 years old reach
sizes greater than 100 gm. Their data suggest that the
growth of BPH is initiated probably before the patient is 30
years old and between the ages of 31 and 50 and the doubling
time for prostatic weight may be 4.5 years. Between the
ages of 51 and 70, the doubling time is 10 years and above
70 years of age, it is 100 years (Berry et al, 1984).

CYTOLOGIC ATYPIA (DYSPLASIA)

Fifty-one total prostatectomy specimens for cancer and 51 autopsy prostates were examined for the presence of atypia which was defined as enlargement of columnar cell nuclei in conjunction with preservation of basal cells (Oyasu et al, 1986). Atypical prostatic hyperplasia was found more frequently in prostatectomy specimens (48 of 51 cases) than in autopsy specimens (14 of 37 cases) after exclusion of cancer associated cases. The atypical prostatic hyperplasia was severe in 42 of the 48 prostatectomy specimens but in only 3 of the 14 autopsy specimens. The distribution of atypical prostatic hyperplasia was similar to that of carcinoma. It was located at sites separate from the carcinoma as well as in contiguous areas (Oyasu et al, 1986).

Foci of cytologic atypia with some of the histologic features of malignancy were sought in ductal and acinar lining epithelia from 100 serially blocked prostates with adenocarcinoma and 100 benign prostates obtained at autopsy (McNeal et al, 1986). Deviations from normal epithelium were regarded grade 1 dysplasia if there were increases in nuclear size, anisokaryosis, and irregularity of nuclear spacing. Grade 2 dysplasia was defined as increased nuclear chromatin in addition to nuclear enlargement, anisokaryosis, and prominent nucleoli in only a few nucleoli. Grade 3 dysplasia was defined as the presence of large prominent eosinophilic nucleoli in the majority of cells. Nuclear hyperchromatism was similar to that seen in grade 2, but chromatin margination at the nuclear membrane was more prominent and present in most nuclei. Eighty-two prostates with carcinoma and 43 benign prostates contained foci of dysplasia. The severity (grade) and extent of the dysplasia were greater in the prostates with carcinoma. Grade 3 dysplasia was found in 33% of the prostates with cancer but in only 4% of the benign prostates. The frequency of multiple independent invasive carcinomas was high among prostates with multiple foci of dysplasia. The authors concluded that dysplasia is probably a direct biologic precursor of prostatic carcinoma and may be the antecedent lesion in the majority of prostatic cancers (McNeal et al, 1986).

In another study, the frequency of atypical hyperplasia in prostate glands without carcinoma was only 2.8%. However, the frequency of atypical hyperplasia in glands with carcinoma was 49.4%. Increasing cytologic atypia was associated with increased tritiated thymidine uptake (Helpap, 1980). Similar criteria were used by these workers in

Dusseldorf and they concluded that the finding of atypical hyperplasia meant that a potentially malignant transformation of the gland had occurred and/or that an already manifest carcinoma may exist in parts of the gland not sampled.

If the data from these three papers are representative and if 25% of all men age 50 to 80 have carcinoma, it would appear that the finding of dysplasia in an older man carries a risk of coincidental or subsequent carcinoma of at least 75%. If he also has a suspicious lesion in the peripheral zone by ultrasonography, the risk of carcinoma must be over 80%.

ADENOCARCINOMA - SITE

The vast majority of typical microacinar carcinomas arise in the peripheral zone:

Fifty percent of the volume of the glandular tissue of the peripheral zone is contained in a shell extending 3 1/3 mm in from the capsule (McNeal, 1969). Sixty-six percent of small carcinomas arose within that zone. Clear-cut premalignant changes were found in benign epithelium near areas of carcinoma and direct transitions could often be demonstrated. Furthermore, the concept of histologically identical but biologically different classes of carcinoma (i.e. latent carcinoma) was not supported. It seemed more reasonable to explain the observations on the basis of a logarithmic growth curve. Biologic malignant potential correlated with tumor size and a progressive loss in differentiation. The capacity for distant metastases appeared to be limited to tumors which are well over 1 cc in volume (McNeal, 1969).

In a study of 208 prostates, Mostofi and Price found neoplasm only in the peripheral zone in 94 and in both the peripheral zone and the central zone in 109. In only one case was the tumor apparently central without peripheral zone involvement. In four, the location could not be ascertained (Mostofi et al, 1973).

ADENOCARCINOMA - GRADE

Three parameters were identified as being prognostically significant in patients with single architectural patterns (formations) in their tumors: nuclear anaplasia, architecture (glands), and mitoses if present. The parameters shown to be of importance for the prognosis in patients whose tumors have single formations also have signi-

ficant influence in patients whose tumors have multiple formations. The worst formation determines prognosis but patients with poorly differentiated tumors do significantly
worse if the tumor is homogeneous. The presence of better
differentiated formations improves the prognosis of the
worst formations (Schroeder et al, 1985). Multivariate analysis of the three independent parameters identified five
separate prognostically different groups (Schroeder et al,
1985).

In a study which correlated the Gleason histologic
grade between biopsy and prostatectomy specimens, the authors found that the Gleason score assigned to the biopsy
specimen was identical to that of the prostatectomy specimen
in 51% of cases, greater than that of the prostatectomy
specimens in 4% and less than that of the prostatectomy
specimens in 45% (Mills et al, 1986). They concluded that
prostatic biopsy should be repeated when the initial diagnosis of adenocarcinoma is based on only limited quantities
of neoplastic tissue with a low Gleason score if management
decisions will be influenced by a true Gleason score of the
tumor. However, another study concluded that the final
Gleason score from the total prostatectomy specimen could be
predicted from the biopsy tissue with reasonably good accuracy (Babaian et al, 1985).

In another study of the accuracy of diagnostic biopsy
specimens in predicting tumor grade by Gleason's classification of radical prostatectomy specimens, the sum of the
Gleason's primary and secondary pattern was within one grade
in all of 115 patients except for 32 cases. The discrepancy
was two grades in 25 patients and three grades in seven.
Nineteen lesions were upgraded and six downgraded. The diagnostic biopsy predicted the grade of the primary tumor in
72% of cases (Garnett et al 1984).

The Gleason grade gave long-term prognostic information
independent of stage with a direct correlation between the
Gleason grade and the cancer death rate index in eighty-two
patients with carcinoma who were followed to death (Sogani
et al, 1985). Furthermore, the sum of the clinical stage
plus the Gleason grade was a more significant prognostic
factor than either stage or grade alone. Gaeta et al described a new measure, the sum of the glandular and nuclear
grades, and found it to be superior to the previously reported maximum of the two grades of the National Prostate
Cancer Treatment Group (Gaeta et al, 1986). However, the
Gleason score was found to be superior to the new measure.

In 1980, Gaeta et al described a combined histologic and cytologic grading system which demonstrated significant correlation with stage at the time of initial diagnosis and mortality rates for each grade group (Gaeta et al, 1980).

In another study, Myers and associates discovered that when nucleoli were prominent or intermediate, the mean interval between initial operative therapy and clinical recurrence was shorter than in a group of patients in which the nuclei were judged to be not prominent (Myers et al, 1982).

Sharkey et al used point-counting and 100 x magnification and divided neoplastic cells into differentiated, meaning the cells lined a gland-like space and contained a nucleus that was polarized away from the lumen and undifferentiated defined as all other neoplastic cells. The percentage of neoplastic cells which were differentiating was 71% in stage A, 59% in stage B, 33% in stage C and 28% in stage D (Sharkey et al, 1984).

A study of four major systems for the histologic grading of primary prostatic cancer was presented by Murphy and Whitmore. The use of the Gleason system alone or in conjunction with other systems was encouraged. It appeared to be definable, reproducible, reasonably simple, and it had clinical relevance as judged by correlations with patient survival.

Flow cytometry has been used to assess tumor cell heterogeneity and the grading of human prostatic cancer. A flow cytometric grading index was established based on the mean and variance in perpendicular and forward light scatter. The index has allowed for the accurate prediction of the ultimate pathologic stage in seven human prostatic cancers obtained at the time of radical retropubic prostatectomy and lymph node dissection. Two patients with high flow cytometric index values had seminal vesicle invasion and capsular penetration by prostatic cancer. Four with intermediate index values had capsular penetration only. A patient with a low index value had a small cancer confined totally to the surgical specimen (Benson et al, 1986).

Frankfurt et al studied the relationship between DNA ploidy, glandular differentiation and tumor spread. DNA ploidy was evaluated by flow cytometry for 45 prostate carcinomas. Twenty tumors contained a distinct aneuploid stem line. All 11 tumors confined to the prostate gland (pathological stage B) were diploid. The frequency of aneuploidy increased with advancing stage and most tumors with distant

metastases were aneuploid. One-third of tumors with a
Gleason score of 5 to 6 were aneuploid whereas over 70% of
poorly differentiated tumors with a Gleason score of 9 to 10
were aneuploid. Among diploid tumors, 46% were localized
carcinomas (stage B), 36% were characterized by invasion
outside the prostate (stage C), and 18% formed pelvic nodal
or distant metastases (stage D1 and D2). Only 7.1% of diploid tumors with a Gleason score of 5 to 6 formed metastases, but 80% of aneuploid tumors with a higher Gleason
score (7 to 10) formed metastases. Diploid tumors with
higher Gleason scores and aneuploid tumors with lower
Gleason scores had intermediate frequencies of metastases.
Aneuploid stem lines in prostate carcinomas were associated
with tumors that had spread outside the prostate gland or
metastasized (Frankfurt et al, 1985).

ADENOCARCINOMA - STAGE

The June 1986 draft of the TNM Clinical Classification
from the Task Force on Urologic Sites of the American Joint
Committee on Cancer was provided by Dr. G.M. Farrow, written
communication 1986.

T- Primary Tumour

TX   Primary tumour cannot be assessed
T0   No evidence of primary tumour
T1   Tumour is incidental histological finding
      T1a   Not more than three microscopic foci of carci-
             noma
      T1b   More than three microscopic foci of carcinoma
T2   Tumour present clinically or grossly limited to the
      gland
      T2a   Tumour 1.5 cm or less in greatest dimension
             with normal tissue on at least three sides
      T2b   Tumour more than 1.5 cm in greatest dimension
             or in more than one lobe
T3   Tumour invades into the prostatic apex or into or be-
      yond the prostatic capsule or bladder neck or seminal
      vesical, but is not fixed.
T4   Tumour is fixed or invades adjacent structures other
      than those listed in T3.

G-Histopathological Grading

GX   Grade of differentiation cannot be assessed
G1   Well differentiated, slight anaplasia
G2   Moderately differentiated, moderate anaplasia
G3-4 Poorly differentiated-undifferentiated, marked ana-
      plasia
Either anaplasia or pattern type of grading method may be
used.

Stage Grouping

Stage 0	T1a	N0	M0	G1
	T2a	N0	M0	G1
Stage I	T1a	N0	M0	G2-4
	T2a	N0	M0	G2-4
Stage II	T1b	N0	M0	Any G
	T2b	N0	M0	Any G
Stage III	T3	N0	M0	Any G
Stage IV	T4	N0	M0	Any G
	Any T	N1,2,3	M0	Any G
	Any T	Any N	M1	Any G

It is apparent that Stage 0 is separated from Stage 1 based
on the histologic grade, Stage 1 is separated from Stage 2
based on the volume of neoplasm, and that T1a and T1b are
the primary tumor designations used when the neoplasm is unsuspected, a so-called incidental finding. T2a and T2b represent small and larger tumors which are clinically evident on physical examination.

So-called Incidental Carcinoma

Opinion is divided as to the appropriate handling of
transurethral resection (TUR) specimens for the detection of
unsuspected carcinomas, see below.

In one study all stage A2 prostatic carcinomas were detected by histologic examination of 6 g of randomly selected
chips. Although additional tumors were detected in direct
proportion to the amount of tissue examined, they were
small, well differentiated, stage A1 lesions. Histologic
sampling of 12 g of randomly selected prostatic chips detected almost 90% of incidental carcinomas including all
clinically significant neoplasms (Murphy et al, 1986).

To achieve a 95% probability of detecting carcinoma in
TUR specimens, a minimum of 95% of the fragments must be examined if one fragment contains a carcinoma, 63.1% of the

fragments if three contain carcinoma, and 25.8% of the fragments if 10 contain carcinoma (Moore et al, 1986).

Eight Hundred and fifty routine prostatectomy specimens
were examined by placing all of the tissue in blocks for
complete microscopic examination. Of these specimens, 711
were obtained from patients in whom cancer had not been diagnosed previously; 61 cancers were found in this group with
49 of these cancers from glands that had not been considered
questionable on clinical examination. For optimal, partial
sampling of transurethral prostatectomy specimens, five
blocks should be submitted; this method is economical and
will detect approximately 90% of cancers including all those
consisting predominantly of Gleason pattern 4 or 5, all progressive cancers, and all cancers identified clinically as
stage 3 or 4. The detection of all focal cancers probably
requires the examination of all tissue but such detection
may be unimportant to the patient's prognosis (Vollmer,
1986).

Of 53 patients, 18 had adenocarcinoma and 35 benign
disease. A mathematical analysis evaluating the probability
of including a carcinoma when different numbers of blocks
were processed was performed. The analysis showed that when
a patient had clinically malignant disease, the probability
of finding carcinoma by the processing of one block was
100%. However, if the patient had a clinically benign diagnosis, a 98% probability of finding the neoplasm was first
reached by the processing of eight blocks, if such an amount
of material was available (Garborg et al, 1985).

Forty-two patients with stage A prostatic adenocarcinoma on initial TUR (defined as tumor of low grade and low
volume-less than 5% of the specimen or less than 3 foci) had
repeat TUR and/or biopsy. In 24 patients who underwent both
procedures, residual carcinoma was identified by TUR in six
and by transperineal needle biopsy in one. Thirty-two patients had no residual carcinoma. Of the 10 with residual
carcinoma, five underwent radical prostatectomy with pelvic
lymphadenectomy, one had interstitial irradiation with pelvic lymphadenectomy and one had pelvic lymphadenectomy only. No lymph nodal metastases were detected. Persistent
carcinoma confined to the prostate was noted in all five
patients who had a radical prostatectomy and three of these
tumors were upstaged because of a higher grade and/or volume. The authors believe that residual carcinoma cannot be
assessed accurately with transperineal needle biopsy
(Carroll et al, 1985).

Of 86 patients with stage A1 in whom additional prostatic tissue was available because of repeat TUR or radical prostatectomy, only six patients were found to have diffuse cancer in the remaining prostatic tissue. Therefore, it appeared that the classification of patients into stage A1 or stage A2 was generally accurate when based upon the findings from the initial TUR alone. Repeat TUR did not appear to contribute significantly to the accuracy of staging (Parfitt et al, 1983).

Following the discovery of incidental adenocarcinoma of the prostate, repeat TUR showed no tumor in 71%, stage A1 in 20%, and stage A2 in 9% (Sonda et al, 1984).

NATURAL HISTORY

McNeal and his group have studied the patterns of progression in prostate cancer. Tumor volume was related to metastasis, seminal vesicle invasion, capsular invasion, and histologic differentiation in a series of 100 unselected prostates with carcinoma removed at necropsy and 38 removed at radical prostatectomy. In both series, metastases were associated only with tumors larger than 4 ml, a volume attained by only 13% of the necropsy tumors. Loss of differentiation strongly correlated with tumor volume and only tumors of Gleason grade 4 or 5 metastasized. Among 56 tumors under 0.46 ml volume in which capsular invasion could be assessed, one case showed a single microscopic focus of carcinoma which extended through the capsule. Three other cases showed foci of neoplasm within but not through the capsule. Among 33 evaluable tumors larger than 0.46 ml, seventeen showed penetration through the capsule and eight showed invasion not quite through the capsule. Furthermore, the extent of the surface area of complete capsular penetration correlated with tumor volume, seminal vesicle invasion and metastatic disease. The authors concluded that the natural history of prostate cancer is highly predictable: the capacity to metastasize probably develops only in tumors which have grown much larger than 1 ml and acquired poorly differentiated areas as a manifestation of tumor progression. The low proportion of metastatic disease is explained by the large proportion of small volume tumors (McNeal et al, 1986). It would appear that the great majority of prostate cancers are at least moderately differentiated at first and subsequently lose differentiation. Precise determination of volume and capsular invasion should improve the estimation of prognosis in the individual patient. The highest categories of either volume or capsular penetration identified the cases with metastases at least as accurately as did the presence of seminal vesicle invasion. The nine metastatic carcinomas from both series all had either a primary or secondary Gleason grade of 4. However, poor differentiation became prevalent in a volume range considerably below that at which metastases was first seen and in the necropsy series 5% of tumors under 0.46 ml were grade 4. This suggests that grade 4 tumors may be a heterogeneous group in terms of their biological malignant potential.

Pontes and co-workers studied 54 radical prostatectomy specimens. In patients with clinical stages A2 and B1, pathologic findings were in accord in most patients (11 of 14). However, only three of 40 patients with clinical stage B2 tumor had pathological stage B2 disease. Seventy-two percent of the tumors were bilateral. Microscopic involvement of the capsule did not appear to influence lymph node invasion since only one of 27 patients with microscopic capsular involvement had pelvic lymph nodal metastases. However, nine of 13 patients with seminal vesicle involvement had pelvic lymph nodal metastases. The addition of flow cytometry to the Gleason score improved the predictive value of the histologic grade in higher stage lesions (Pontes et al, 1985). A comparison of the histologic findings by Gleason grade between the needle biopsy in the final pathological specimen revealed that biopsies undergraded the tumor in 24 cases (45%) and overgraded in two.

Kuban and associates found that there was no evidence that TUR of the prostate gland caused metastasis of the neoplasm to bone. One Hundred of 169 patients with a minimum of four year follow up had transurethral resection before treatment. The incidence of bony metastases increased progressively with decreasing tumor differentiation and advancing tumor stage (Kuban et al, 1985).

Smith and Middleton studied the implications of the volume of lymph nodal metastases in patients with adenocarcinoma of the prostate. Of the patients with grossly evident lymph nodal disease, 15% survived five years without progression compared to 27% of patients with microscopic involvement of more than one node and 44% with a single positive node. In addition, 52% of patients with grossly evident disease died of prostatic cancer within five years compared to 37% with multiple microscopic lymph nodal involvement and 28% with involvement of a single lymph node (Smith et al, 1985).

Plesnicar studied the course of metastatic disease originating from carcinoma of the prostate. Bone metastases were found to be osteoblastic or both osteoblastic and osteolytic. In patients with solely osteoblastic bone metastases, the lesions were hormone sensitive and long-lasting remissions could be obtained. The development of osteolytic bone lesions was usually accompanied by the recurrence of the primary tumor, and the appearance of metastases in other sites such as lymph nodes and lungs. The bone metastases became resistant to hormonal manipulation and short remissions were obtained with chemotherapy. The course of the terminal period was faster with shorter survival times (Plesnicar, 1985).

TUMOR MARKERS

The relative reliability of prostate-specific antigen (PSA), prostatic acid phosphatase (PAP), acid phosphatase, bone alkaline phosphatase (BAP), and total alkaline phosphatase have been evaluated in 79 patients with prostate cancer stages B2 to D1 and 51 patients with stage D2 disease. For patients with stage D2 disease, only serial elevated levels of PSA, BAP, and PAP are prognostically reliable. Furthermore, after adjustment for the effect of PSA, no other marker is significantly related to the risk of disease progression. Only elevated levels of serial PSA and PAP are prognostically significant in patients with stages B2 to D1 disease (Killian et al, 1986; Chu et al, 1986). Patients with early stage disease can be reliably followed with the use of PSA and PAP, not only for detection of disease progression when markers are elevated, but also for prediction of a six months favorable prognosis when PSA levels are within a normal reference range. A good prognosis may be indicated in patients with advanced stage disease when PSA, BAP, and PAP levels are within a normal reference limit. Conversely, in patients with advanced disease, if the levels of PSA, BAP, and PAP are elevated, an unfavorable prognosis should be anticipated (Killian et al, 1986).

Seamonds et al measured PSA and PAP in patients with prostate cancer, benign prostatic hypertrophy (BPH) and prostatitis. PSA was more sensitive than PAP for the detection of newly diagnosed cancer and relapses. Both were highly specific. However, PSA was found to be more sensitive for monitoring therapy since it usually rose before PAP and always proceeded clinical signs of relapse. PSA was found to be elevated more frequently than PAP in some pa-

tients with BPH and prostatitis. The authors speculated
that patients with elevated serum PSA and normal PAP may
fall into a high risk subpopulation which may have early
prostate cancer or precancerous conditions not usually detectable by current techniques. Five of seven patients with
A1 disease had an elevated PSA whereas none had elevated
PAP. All 33 patients with stage A2 through D prostate
cancer had elevated PSA; 24 had an elevated serum PAP. PAP
in combination with PSA may serve as a useful adjunct for
differential diagnosis and confirmation of advanced stage
prostate cancer (Seamonds et al, 1986). Because BPH patients who are subsequently diagnosed as having carcinoma of
the prostate gland had abnormal serum PSA, the authors believe that the finding of an abnormal serum PSA in a BPH
patient may be prove to be useful in distinguishing those
who may have early carcinoma or atypical hyperplasia. Furthermore, the authors believe that baseline PSA levels on
all patients who are having transurethral resection or biopsy of the prostate may be helpful to alert the pathologist
to look more closely for the possible presence of prostate
cancer or focal atypia and in assessing the efficacy of subsequent therapy. Those with lower pretreatment levels of
serum PSA tend to survive longer than those with higher levels.

OTHER CARCINOMAS

So-called endometrioid carcinomas account for 1% of all
carcinomas (Brooks et al, 1986 and Epstein et al, 1986).
These neoplasms are positive for PSA and PAP by histochemistry (Bostwick et al, 1985; Epstein et al, 1986). Mucinous
adenocarcinomas of the prostate gland are also positive for
PSA and/or PAP by histochemistry (Epstein et al, 1985 and
Odom et al, 1986).

REFERENCES

Babaian RJ, Grunow WA (1985). Reliability of Gleason grading system in comparing prostate biopsies with total prostatectomy specimens. Urology Jun;25(6):564-7.
Benson MC, Walsh PC (1986). The application of flow cytometry to the assessment of tumor cell heterogeneity and
  the grading of human prostatic cancer: preliminary results. J Urol June;135(6):1194-1198.
Berry SJ, Coffey DS, Walsh PC, Ewing LL (1984). The development of human benign prostatic hyperplasia with age. J
  Urol Sep;132(3):474-9.

Bostwick DG, Kindrachuk RW, Rouse RV (1985). Prostatic adenocarcinoma with endometrioid features. Clinical, pathologic, and ultrastructural findings. Am J Surg Pathol
Aug;9(8):595-609.

Bostwick DG, Mann RB (1985). Malignant lymphomas involving
the prostate. A study of 13 cases. Cancer Dec 15;56(12):
2932-8.

Brooks B, Miller GJ (1986). Evaluation of prostatic cancer
histology and grade distribution: experience with the Col-
orado Central Cancer Registry. Prostate 8(2):139-50.

Carroll PR, Leitner TC, Yen TS, Watson RA, Williams RD
(1985). Incidental carcinoma of the prostate: significance of staging transurethral resection. J Urol May;
133(5):811-4.

Chu TM, Murphy GP (1986). What's new in tumor markers for
prostate cancer? Urology June;27(6):487-491.

Epstein JI, Lieberman PH (1985). Mucinous adenocarcinoma of
the prostate gland. Am J Surg Pathol Apr;9(4):299-308.

Epstein JI, Woodruff JM (1986). Adenocarcinoma of the prostate with endometrioid features. A light microscopic and
immunohistochemical study of ten cases. Cancer Jan 1;57
(1):111-9.

Frankfurt OS, Chin JL, Englander LS, Greco WR, Pontes JE,
Rustum YM (1985). Relationship between DNA ploidy, glandular differentiation, and tumor spread in human prostate
cancer. Cancer Res Mar;45(3):1418-23.

Gaeta JF, Asirwatham JE, Miller G, Murphy GP (1980). Histologic grading of primary prostatic cancer: A new approach to an old problem. J Urol 123:689-93.

Gaeta JF, Englander LC, Murphy GP (1986). Comparative evaluation of National Prostatic Cancer Treatment Group and
Gleason systems for pathologic grading of primary prostatic cancer. Urology Apr;27(4):306-8.

Garborg I, Eide TJ (1985). The probability of overlooking
prostatic cancer in transurethrally resected material when
different embedding practices are followed. Acta Pathol
Microbiol Immunol Scand (A) Sep;93(5):205-8.

Garnett JE, Oyasu R, Grayhack JT (1984). The accuracy of
diagnostic biopsy specimens in predicting tumor grades by
Gleason's classification of radical prostatectomy specimens. J Urol Apr;131(4):690-3.

Helpap B (1980). The biological significance of atypical
hyperplasia of prostate. Virchows Arch A Path Anat and
Histol 387:307-17.

Killian CS, Emrich LJ, Vargas FP, Yang N, Wang MC, Priore
RL, Murphy GP, Chu TM (1986). Relative reliability of

five serially measured markers for prognosis of progression in prostate cancer. JNCI 76:179-185.

Kuban DA, el-Mahdi AM, Schellhammer PF, Babb TJ (1985). The effect of transurethral prostatic resection on the incidence of osseous prostatic metastasis. Cancer Aug 15;56 (4):961-4.

McNeal JE (1984). Anatomy of the prostate and morphogenesis of BPH. Prog Clin Biol Res 145:27-53.

McNeal JE (1969). Origin and development of carcinoma in the prostate. Cancer Jan;23:24-34.

McNeal JE (1968). Regional morphology and pathology of the prostate. Am J Clin Path 49:347-357.

McNeal JE, Bostwick DG (1984). Anatomy of the prostatic urethra (letter); JAMA Feb 17;251(7):890-1.

McNeal JE, Bostwick DG (1986). Intraductal dysplasia: a premalignant lesion of the prostate. Hum Pathol Jan;17 (1):64-71.

McNeal JE, Bostwick DG, Kindrachuk RA, Redwine EA, Freiha FS, Stamey TA (1986). Patterns of progression in prostate cancer. Lancet Jan 11;1(8472):60-3.

Mills SE, Fowler JE Jr (1986). Gleason histologic grading of prostatic carcinoma. Correlations between biopsy and prostatectomy specimens. Cancer Jan 15;57(2):346-9.

Moore GH, Lawshe B, Murphy J (1986). Diagnosis of adenocarcinoma in transurethral resectates of the prostate gland. Am J Surg Pathol Mar;10(3):165-9.

Mostofi FK, Price EB Jr (1973). Tumors of the male genital system. Atlas of Tumor Pathol, Second Series, Fascicle 8, AFIP Washington, DC.

Murphy WM, Dean PJ, Brasfield JA, Tatum L (1986). Incidental carcinoma of the prostate. How much sampling is adequate? Am J Surg Pathol Mar;10(3):170-4.

Myers RP, Neves RJ, Farrow GM, Utz DC (1982). Nucleolar grading of prostatic adenocarcinoma: light microscopic correlation with disease progression. Prostate 3:423-432.

Odom DG, Donatucci CF, Deshon GE (1986). Mucinous Adenocarcinoma of the Prostate. Hum Pathol 17:863-865.

Oyasu R, Bahnson RR, Nowels K, Garnett JE (1986). Cytologic atypia in the prostate gland: frequency, distribution and possible relevance to carcinoma. J Urol May;135(5):959-62.

Parfitt HE, Smith JA, Gliedman JB, Middleton RG (1983). Accuracy of staging in A1 Carcinoma of the prostate. Cancer 51:2346-50.

Plesnicar S (1985). The course of metastatic disease originating from carcinoma of the prostate. Clin Exp Metastasis Apr-Jun;3(2):103-10.

Pontes JE, Wajsman Z, Huben RP, Wolf RM, Englander LS (1985). Prognostic factors in localized prostatic carcinoma. J Urol Dec;134(6):1137-9.

Schroeder FH, Blom JH, Hop WC, Mostofi FK (1985). Grading of prostatic cancer: An analysis of the prognostic significance of single characteristics. Prostate 6(1):81-100.

Schroeder FH, Blom JH, Hop WC, Mostofi FK (1985). Grading of prostatic cancer: II. The prognostic significance of the presence of multiple architectural patterns. Prostate 6(4):403-15.

Schroeder FH, Hop WC, Blom JH, Mostofi FK (1985). Grading of prostatic cancer: III. Multivariate analysis of prognostic parameters. Prostate 7(1):13-20.

Seamonds B, Yang N, Anderson K, Whitaker B, Shaw LM, Bollinger JR (1986). Evaluation of prostate-specific antigen and prostatic acid phosphatase as prostate cancer markers. Accepted by Urology.

Sharkey FE, Dusenbery DM, Moyer JE, Barry JD (1984). Correlation between stage and grade in prostatic adenocarcinoma: a morphometric study. J Urol Sep;132(3):602-5.

Smith JA Jr., Middleton RG (1985). Implications of volume of nodal metastasis in patients with adenocarcinoma of the prostate. J Urol Apr;133(4):617-9.

Sogani PC, Israel A, Lieberman PH, Lesser ML, Whitmore WF Jr (1985). Gleason grading of prostate cancer: a predictor of survival. Urology Mar;25(3):223-7.

Sonda LP, Grossman HB, MacGregor RJ, Gikas PW (1984). Incidental adenocarcinoma of the prostate: the role of repeat transurethral resection in staging. Prostate 5(2):141-6.

Tisell LE, Salander H (1984). Anatomy of the human prostate and its three paired lobes. Prog Clin Biol Res 145:55-65.

Vollmer RT (1986). Prostate cancer and chip specimens: complete versus partial sampling. Hum Pathol Mar;17(3):285-90.

The Use of Transrectal Ultrasound in the Diagnosis and
Management of Prostate Cancer, pages 31–48
© 1987 Alan R. Liss, Inc.

PERTINENT PHYSICS OF AN OPTIMAL EXAMINATION

Albert Goldstein Ph.D.

Depts of Ob/Gyn and Radiology
Wayne State University
Detroit, Michigan 48201

Diagnostic ultrasound has become an important imaging
modality for the visualization of many internal soft tissue
structures. It is the imaging modality of choice in Ob/Gyn
examinations, cardiac studies and assessment of the peripheral vascular system. It is also used extensively for imaging the abdominal organs, the neonatal brain, the testes
and many other soft tissue organs. Recently, the technolog-
ical advances that have been made in the development of so
called "small parts" scanners (which are used to obtained
detailed images of small regions located close to the skin
surface) have been extended to the use of intracorporial
probes which penetrate into the body through natural ori-
fices (the rectum, esophagus, vaginal etc.) or through in-
cisions made during surgical procedures and give high quality ultrasound images of important anatomy which is located
at great depths from the skin surface.

Transrectal ultrasonic imaging of the prostate is one
such area that is revolutionizing the diagnosis and treatment of prostatic disease. It is the purpose of this chapter to acquaint the reader with the fundamentals of ultrasound imaging and to demonstrate the important imaging improvements gained with the use of transrectal ultrasonic
probes. Also, some important technical factors, under the
operator's control, which affect diagnostic image quality
will be discussed.

Figure 1(a) demonstrates the method of performing a
standard ultrasound contact scan to obtain an image of the
prostate gland. The ultrasound transducer is the device

which is used to generate the output ultrasound pulse (high
frequency sound waves) and to also receive the echoes generated by the output pulse as it travels down into the

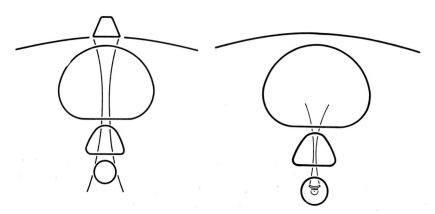

Figure 1. Contact and Transrectal Scans of Prostate
In contact scanning, (a) on left, the transducer beam
must penetrate through the filled urinary bladder to
the triangular prostate gland. In transrectal scanning, (b) on right, the side-looking transducer (on
the end of a cylindrical probe) is scanning the
adjacent prostate gland.

body's soft tissues. The transducer is moved on the skin
surface looking down into the body. Even though it is in
constant "contact" with the skin surface, a thin layer of
gel must be used to acoustically couple the transducer to
the body so that the ultrasound output pulse can leave the
transducer and enter the body and at a later time the scattered echoes can reenter the transducer. The main reason
for the need of the gel is to eliminate any air which may
become trapped between the transducer and the skin. Ultrasound energy reflects of off an air interface and, thus,
will not be able to penetrate into the patient. Any air
bubbles inside of the body similarly reflect the ultrasound
and lead to acoustic shadows which degrade the image's diagnostic potential.

In Figure 1(a) the transducer is positioned over the filled urinary bladder which is used as a convenient acoustic window to the posterior prostate gland. The transducer beam pattern (which is the path in the tissue of the output ultrasound pulse) is shown. As the output pulse travels down the beam pattern some of its energy scatterers off of soft tissue structures and returns to the transducer in the form of an ultrasonic echo. The ultrasound equipment measures the time it takes for the echoes to return to the transducer and from this measured travel time and the known speed of sound calculates the depth of the tissue scatterers. Since the equipment also "knows" the direction of the transducer beam pattern inside of the patient, it can generate an image of the patient's soft tissue with all of the soft tissue reflectors placed in their correct anatomical positions. The amplitude of the received echoes is encoded in the image using a gray scale. The shade of gray used to register a reflector's position indicates its received echo amplitude. Many years of experience with gray scale ultrasound images have shown that the lower amplitude shades of gray in the image are sometimes the most important in identifying small focal lesions or the presence of diffuse disease.

The contact scan transducer used to image the prostate is the one used for most ultrasound examinations and has been designed as a compromise between tissue penetration and good image quality at various depths in the ultrasound images. In Figure 1(a), the prostate is seen at the lower depths of the image where the focussed beam pattern is beginning to widen.

Figure 1(b) demonstrates a transrectal scan of the prostate using a transducer mounted on a rectal probe. Since the prostate is adjacent to the rectum a smaller transducer with a much narrower beam pattern can be used to image the prostate gland. The transducer is mounted on a rectal probe and the rectal probe is covered by a condum. After the probe has been inserted into the rectum, the condum is fill with water. The water serves several purposes. It is the acoustic coupling medium between the transducer and the patient permitting the ultrasound energy to travel between the two. The water filled condum also pushes aside any air in the rectum preventing these air pockets from causing deleterious acoustic shadows in the prostatic image. (Bits of fecal matter which become trapped between the condum and the rectal wall can also cause shadows in the image and should be avoided by proper preparation of the patient.) Finally, the liquid filled condum compresses the prostate which sometimes improves the ultrasound image quality.

TRANSRECTAL SCAN PLANES

Two types of transrectal ultrasound probes are used: the transaxial side-looking transducer and the linear array. The transaxial probe usually has a single element transducer (disk shaped and focussed) which is mounted so that its beam pattern is perpendicular to the axis of the probe (side-looking). A small motor is used to slowly rotate the transducer so that its beam sweeps out a scan plane which is perpendicular to the axes of the probe and rectum. A series of transaxial (or axial) scan planes is shown in Figure 2(a). They were acquired by moving the probe into the rectum in equal steps between scans.

TRANSAXIAL SCAN PLANES

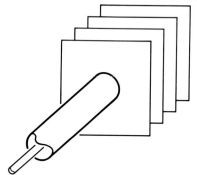

SAGITTAL SCAN PLANES

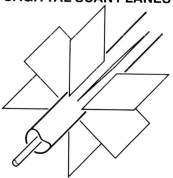

Figure 2. Transrectal Scan Planes
In (a) on left, a side-looking single element transducer is rotated about the rectal probe axis and generates transaxial scan planes perpendicular to the axis of the rectum. In (b) on right, a linear array transducer is mounted along the axis of the rectal probe. The sagittal scan plane of the linear array moves outward from the axis of the rectum and can be positioned at any orientation by the operator.

The other type of transducer is a linear array which is a more complicated structure than the single element transducer. It is composed of small individual elements some as tiny as 6 thousands of an inch across. The individual elements are arranged in a linear array pattern. Complex electronic circuits are used to control the firing of this transducer and the reception of the returning echoes. Sequentially along the array small groups of elements are used to transmit and receive echoes. The parallel beam patterns from these groups forms a rectangular scan plane in the patient. Since the linear array is mounted with its axis parallel to the probe axis, its scan plane contains the rectum axis (sagittal scan plane) and the operator can chose different scan plane orientations by simply rotating the probe as demonstrated in Figure 2(b). Thus, the two different transducers used in ultrasonic prostate imaging produce scan planes or images from two different orientations orthogonal to each other. The transaxial view is more convenient for initial surveys of the prostate and permits a left - right comparison of the gland's internal anatomy. The sagittal view is more convenient in the ultrasound guided needle procedures used in biopsy and therapy.

ADVANTAGES OF TRANSRECTAL SCANNING

As indicated in Figures 1(a) and 1(b), the difference between contact scans and transrectal scans of the prostate is the proximity of the transducer to the organ. This is a very important factor because it permits higher quality images with finer detail to be made. Three advantages are gained in ultrasonic imaging when the transducer is close to the tissue structure of interest: narrower beam patterns, higher frequencies can be used and better line density in the images.

Beam Pattern

The spatial image detail will be finer (and smaller focal lesion visualized) with narrower transducer beam patterns. The narrow beam pattern is receiving echoes from a smaller volume of tissue and this leads to a more detailed or fine image. So when designing a transducer it is important to have as narrow a beam as possible over as large a range of image depths as possible. However, the rules of optics limit the beam pattern shape that may be attained.

Figures 3(a) and 3(b) demonstrate several of the properties
of focussed transducer beams. The focussed beam is characterized by two parameters: the focal length and the focal
zone. The focal length is the distance between the front
face of the transducer and the depth of the narrowest portion of its beam pattern. This is what focussing means -
concentrating the beam energy at a point a focal length
away from the transducer. The focal zone is the range of
distances (image depths) along the beam pattern where it is
sufficiently narrow to give the best image detail. Each focussed transducer has a focal zone and has its finest image
at the focal zone depths. (Some newer transducers have multiple zone focussing in which electronic focussing is used
to combine the focal zones of several different electronically generated focal lengths of the same transducer in order to have a larger effective total focal zone in the
image.) Figure 3(a) demonstrates one rule concerning focal
zones. For the same diameter and frequency, as the focal
length is made longer the focal zone also increases in
size. So for the typical clinical contact scanning imaging
tasks the best compromise transducer has a large diameter
and a long focal length. The large diameter permits focussing deeper into the body and the long focal length is
used to gain the advantage of a long focal zone. Figure
3(b) demonstrates that for the same frequency and focal

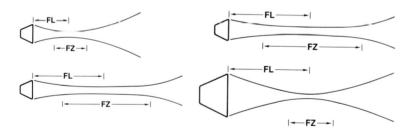

Figure 3. Focussing Principles
In (a) on left we see that the focal zone extent of a
focussed transducer is proportional to its focal
length (for constant diameter and frequency), the
longer the focal length the larger the focal zone. In
(b) on right we see that the focal zone extent of a
focussed transducer is inversely proportional to its
diameter (for constant frequency and focal length).
The larger the diameter the shorter the focal zone.

length the transducer diameter determines the extent of the focal zone. The larger diameter transducer has the shorter focal zone. So when a large diameter transducer is focussed to look at close structures it does so with very fine image detail but over a very limited range of image depths.

Thus, we see the advantage of having the transducer in close proximity to the prostate. It is not necessary to use a large diameter transducer to get deep focussing because we only need to focus close. The smaller diameter, at the focal length required, has a longer focal zone than the larger diameter transducer would have. Also, the beam width in the focal zone will be narrow due to the smaller transducer diameter. Other advantages accrue from the smaller diameter. The received echo amplitude is independent of the transducer diameter (because it is a pressure sensitive device) so there is no reduction in echo signal and smaller transducers are easier to insert into the rectum.

Transducer Frequency

The higher the transducer frequency the shorter the ultrasound waves that are emitted and received. Shorter ultrasound waves give finer image detail so it is always desirable to use the highest frequency possible in ultrasound imaging. However, tissue attenuation (absorption) of the ultrasound is proportional to frequency. As higher frequency transducers are used, the echoes from deep structures get weaker. At the maximum amplifier gain (strength), the frequency and the maximum image depth are inversely proportional. For example, if we use a new transducer with a 40% higher frequency, then the maximum patient depth that can be imaged decreases by 40%.

General purpose contact scanners are equipped with transducers whose frequencies are limited by the large patient depths that must be imaged. Of course, this equipment also has higher frequency transducers available which can give finer images, but these transducers are only used to image shallow soft tissue structures in the body. In contact scanning (Figure 1(a)) a lower frequency transducer (with a larger diameter) would have to be used than in transrectal scanning (Figure 1(b)) because the prostate is much further away. If the prostate is three times further away in the contact scanning case (than in the transrectal scanning case), then the highest frequency that could be used would be three times lower. This results in coarser and much less acceptable images of the prostate. Or, put in other words, the advent of ultrasound transrectal prostate scans lead to much more detailed images of the prostate due to the higher frequencies utilized.

Image Line Density

TRANSAXIAL LINE DENSITY

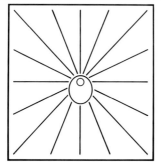

SAGITTAL LINE DENSITY

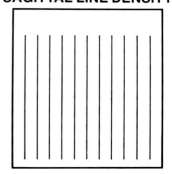

Figure 4. Image Line Density
Since the ultrasound lines in the transaxial view of the prostate ((a) on left) were generated by a rotat- ing transducer, they are radial in nature. Since a linear array transducer generated the image lines, they are all parallel and define a rectangular field of view in the sagittal view ((b) right).

Figures 4(a) and 4(b) demonstrate the image line den- sity in transaxial and sagittal prostate scans. Each image line represents the direction in space of the transducer beam pattern when it transmitted and received ultrasound echoes from tissue. The image detail along the direction of the lines is governed by the transducer frequency and beam pattern. High frequency, small diameter focussed transduc- ers will give fine image detail along the lines. The image detail perpendicular to the lines is simply governed by the line density or number of lines per cm in the patient. (This is similar to the vertical resolution in a TV image which is governed by the density of the horizontal scan lines.)

Modern ultrasound imaging equipment is real-time in nature. The transducer is pulsed rapidly and the received echo information is used to compose image frames which are presented to the viewer at a certain frame rate (number of frames per second). There is always a compromise between the number of lines in the image and the frame rate because of the finite velocity of sound. As shown in Figure 5(a), the transducer cannot send out the next output pulse until

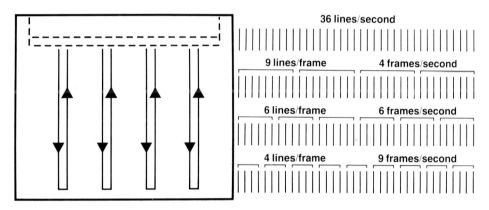

Figure 5. Line Density Considerations
The pulse repetition frequency (number of output pulses per second) is governed by the time it takes for echoes to be received from the maximum image depth as shown in (a) on left. The number of image lines received per second may be divided up into dif-ferent numbers of frames per second with different line densities as shown in (b) on right.

it has received echoes from the tissue at the bottom (furthest from the transducer) of the image. Due to the magnitude of the velocity of sound (1540 meters per sec-ond), this requirement severely limits the number of ultra-sound transmissions per second (each transmission equals one image line). With a real-time image the image lines must be divided up into a certain number of frames per sec-ond. Figure 5(b) illustrates the fictitious case of 36 lines per second being received (the real number is roughly

four to five thousand per second). The 36 lines can be divided up into 4 frames per second, six frames per second or
9 frames per second. At the low frame rates there is a
larger number of lines per frame and the spatial resolution
(fineness of image) is greatest. At the high frame rates
the temporal resolution is greatest and the frame spatial
resolution is the least due to the low number of lines per
frame. In prostatic scanning we are not concerned with following fast tissue motion so that a slow frame rate is chosen with a correspondingly high image line density.

The line density of the magnified transrectal prostatic images is higher than for the contact scanning case
because of two reasons. These are illustrated in Figures
6(a) and 6(b). The first is that the transrectal image has
a smaller field of view in the patient. This magnified
image results in a larger line density in the patient
image. In Figure 6(a) we see the effect of a smaller field
of view for a constant number (four) of lines per frame.
When the field of view is reduced by half (from 12 to 6 cm)
then the four image lines represent more lines per patient
dimension. The second reason is that the smaller field of
view has a smaller image depth so that the pulse repetition
frequency can be increased. As shown in Figure 6(b), when
the image depth is reduced from 12 to 6 cm the number of

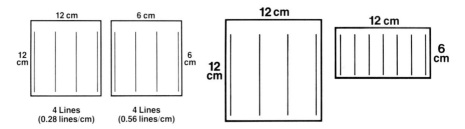

Figure 6. Field of View vs. Line Density
The number of lines per centimeter of patient tissue
depends on the size of the imaged field of view for
the same number of lines in each image as shown in
(a) on left. As the image depth decreases the time
required between transducer output pulses decreases
and the pulse repetition frequency (image lines per
second) increases as shown in (b) on right.

lines per frame (at a constant frame rate) increases by a
factor 2. Putting these two effects together, as shown in
Figure 7, we see that in a magnified image there is a substantial increase in the image line density. Remember that
this is only true if the tissue to be viewed in the magnified image is close to the transducer such as in the case
of transrectal prostatic imaging.

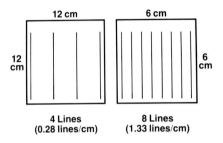

Figure 7. Magnified Image Line Density
Combining the two effects demonstrated in Figures
6(a) and 6(b), we see that there is a substantial increase in image line density for tissue adjacent to
the transducer.

In modern ultrasound equipment the individual image
lines are not usually visible in the image because special
software is used to fill in the image areas between the
lines. However much cosmetic software is used, the tissue
detail perpendicular to the lines-of-sight of the transducer is always determined by the "true" line density in
this direction.

SCANNING PROCEDURES

The rules of optics and common sense dictate some simple procedures that can aid the operator in obtaining the
optimum prostatic images.

Focal Zone Placement

The operator has some control over the placement of
the transducer focal zone in the image. Since the focal

zone is the region of best image detail, it is important to
use this control properly. This is illustrated in Figure
8(a). One possible imaging situation is that the transducer
is moved close to the rectal wall. Then its focal zone
would extend deeper into the body to give better image detail at the far image depths. However, in this case the
prostate's peripheral zone may be close to the rectal wall
and not properly visualized in the image because it is outside of the transducer's focal zone. It would be better
technique for the operator to move the transducer away from
the rectal wall so that its focal zone is moved in closer
to the rectal wall resulting in a more detailed view of the

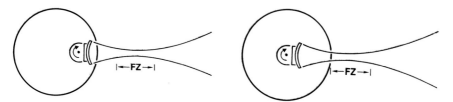

Figure 8. Focal Zone Placement
In (a) on the left, the transducer (mounted on a rectal probe) has been moved close to the rectal wall
giving the best tissue visualization at far image
depths. In (b) on the right, the transducer has been
moved back from the rectal wall in order to obtain
more image detail for tissue close to the rectal
wall.

peripheral zone of the prostate as is shown in Figure 8(b).
So another reason for dilating the rectum with the liquid
filled condum is to permit shifting of the focal zone in
the image.

A simple analogy may help inexperienced operators to
master this concept. In the magnified image consider the
focal zone to be the lens of a magnifying glass connected
to the transducer by a fixed length handle (whose length
defines the focal length). Then to move the magnifying
glass (with its fine image detail) in the image simply move
the transducer position accordingly.

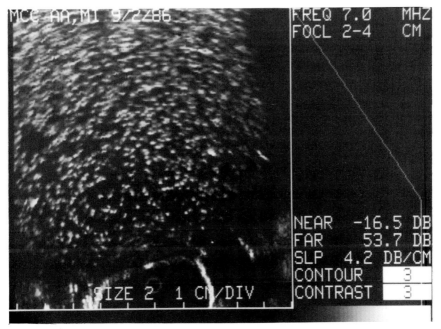

Figure 9(a). Probe Close to Rectal Wall
A new image resolution test object (1) is used to
demonstrate the transducer's 2-4 cm focal zone being
placed at far distances in the image

The effect of moving the focal zone in the image is
dramatically demonstrated in Figures 9(a) and 9(b). In
these figures we see the ultrasound images obtained with
the use of a test object specifically designed to show
image detail (1). The test object consists of an anechoeic
gel into which is placed a uniform dispersion of small
point scatterers. At the image depths of the focal zone the
images of the point reflectors are small and well defined.
At image depths outside of the focal zone the point reflector images are blurred indicating a lack of image detail.
These two images correspond to the situations shown
schematically in Figures 8(a) and 8(b) and clearly demonstrate the importance of proper operator placement of the
focal zone in the prostatic image.

Scan Plane Position

The interval between transaxial or sagittal scan planes affects the ability to detect the presence of small

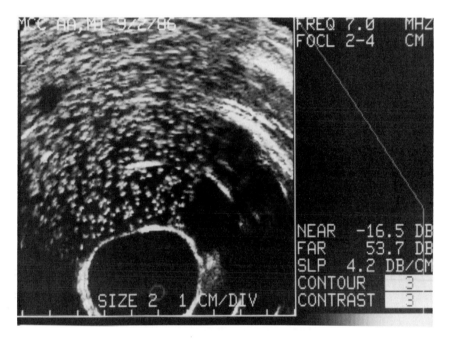

Figure 9(b). Probe Far from Rectal Wall
A new image resolution test object (1) is used to demonstrate the transducer's 2-4 cm focal zone being placed close to the rectal wall for optimum visualization of the peripheral zone.

focal lesions in the prostate. This is illustrated in Figures 10(a) and 10(b) for sets of transaxial and sagittal scan planes. If the interval between transaxial scan planes is equal to the lesion diameter then some lesions which are located midway between the scan planes may be entirely missed in the scan plane images. Similarly, for the case of sagittal scan planes, small lesions which are located far from the rectum can be missed if the angle between scan planes is too large.

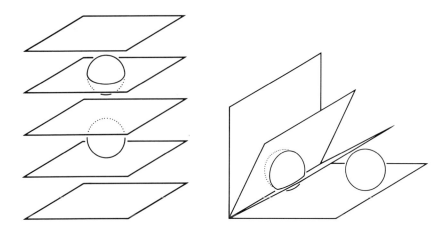

Figure 10. Focal Lesion Detection
The effect of the scan plane locations on focal lesion detection is illustrated for transrectal scans
in (a) on left and sagittal scans in (b) on right. If
the interval between scan planes is equal to the lesion diameter or larger, then it is possible to entirely miss the lesion in the scan plane images.

Fortunately with the use of the real-time imaging
equipment, this potential difficulty can be avoided quite
easily. While viewing the real-time image slowly move the
scan plane. For transaxial scans this means slowly inserting (or removing) the probe. For sagittal scans this means
slowly rotating the probe at the same depth in the rectum.
By slowly moving the probe a large number of adjacent scan
planes can be viewed rapidly and effectively. Video taping
this procedure documents completely the survey of the entire prostate organ. Image hardcopy can then be obtained
for the specific scan planes which demonstrate focal disease or other pathology of interest. It is also possible to
obtain hardcopy from a frozen frame of the video tape.

RESEARCH IN IMAGE OPTIMIZATION

We have been examining the ultrasound equipment imaging parameters in order find ways to improve the quality of
transrectal images. Our initial observations have lead us
to believe that the effect of the transducer frequency on
soft tissue contrast in the image is not completely under-
stood and, in fact, may prove extremely important in tissue
characterization of prostatic pathology. The use of the
frequency as a contrast agent is a new idea in clinical
ultrasound imaging and a potentially important one. Up until the present, clinical scans have been performed with
the limited number of transducer frequencies available and
not much importance has been given to the concept of viewing the tissue structures of interest at different frequencies in order to gain more information.

The role of transducer frequency up until now has been
confined to the concept of spatial resolution. Higher frequencies give better image spatial resolution and, therefore, more image detail. The limits on the frequency used
for imaging have been 1) the stronger tissue attenuation of
the higher frequencies (limiting penetration at high frequencies) and 2) the difficulty of fabricating high frequency real-time multiple element array transducers. As
mentioned above, in transrectal ultrasound imaging the
prostate is adjacent to the transducer so the highest
available frequencies may be utilized to produce good quality images. However, we have found that it may be more ad-
visable to use midrange frequencies in order to maximize
the soft tissue image contrast between the malignant primary lesions in the peripheral zone and the surrounding
normal peripheral zone tissue.

Figure 11 demonstrates some of our experimental evidence. Four scans are shown of an excised prostate gland,
fixed in formalin, at different transducer frequencies.
These scans were obtained with a static scanner (B-Scanner)
and demonstrate the same contrast changes with frequency
that we have also seen using many different real-time scanners. The transducer frequencies are indicated at the lower
right hand corner of the image. Frequencies of 2.25, 3.5,
5.0 and 7.5 MHz were used. As the frequency is increased
the margin of the lesion in the upper left side of the
prostate becomes much better defined in terms of spatial
resolution or detail. The image at 3.5 MHz demonstrates a

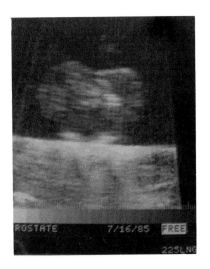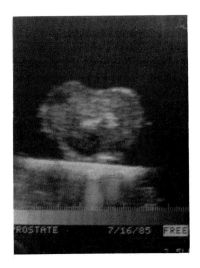
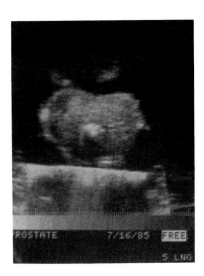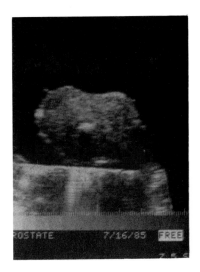

Figure 11. Frequency Dependent Contrast
These four scans of an excised prostate demonstrate
an observed change in lesion contrast with transducer
frequency. See text for details.

hypoechoic lesion with a high degree of image contrast between it and the surrounding normal tissue. However, at the
highest frequency of 7.5 MHz the interior of the lesion is
becoming more echogenic and the image contrast between the
lesion and the surrounding normal tissue has decreased.
Thus, we see a image trade-off between spatial detail and
lesion contrast both of which are governed by the transducer frequency.

We are now in the process of investigating the cause
of this frequency dependent tissue contrast effect to make
certain that it is due to the tissue and not to the
ultrasound equipment. We hope to determine the optimum
frequency to use for transrectal prostatic scanning in
order to enhance our ability to identify small primary
malignant lesions in the peripheral zone.

REFERENCES

1- PIRTO Test Object, RMI Inc. Middleton Wi (608) 831-1188

The Use of Transrectal Ultrasound in the Diagnosis and
Management of Prostate Cancer, pages 49–56
© 1987 Alan R. Liss, Inc.

THE PERFORMANCE OF AN OPTIMAL TRANSRECTAL EXAMINATION OF THE PROSTATE

Richard D. McLeary, M.D.

Department of Radiology, St. Joseph Mercy
Hospital, Ann Arbor, MI 48106

With the development of grey scale image processing, digital scan converters, and higher frequency transducers, it is now possible to obtain information about the inner structure of the prostate gland. However even the most sophisticated equipment is capable of producing horrid images if not correctly operated. The imaging unit; that is, the ultrasonic scanner, sonologist, and patient must all be optimized to obtain the best possible images.

To obtain an optimal examination the patient must be positioned comfortably so that he will not be apt to move during the exam. The patient's rectum should be as clean and empty of air and fecal material as possible. We have had success with the patient self-administering a pre-packaged enema (FLEET ENEMA #1) fifteen minutes before the examination. On the rare occasion that this does not adequately cleanse and empty the rectum it is repeated.

The examination is performed with the patient in the left decubitous, knee-chest position. With the patient in this position any residual gas within the rectum should be outside of the area of interest. If the patient has not had a recent digital rectal examination, one is performed prior to insertion of the transducer. If the patient has any history of anal stricture or fissure the digital exam will allow the operator to determine whether the transducer can be passed into the rectum.

Using a liberal amount of lubricant, the axial transducer is gently inserted into the rectum to a level above the external sphincter. The condom is then filled with the appropriate amount of still water (usually 50cc) and the examination may commence.

All images will be presented in the following fashion uless otherwise noted. The axial images will be shown as viewed form the patient's foot. The right side of the image will be on the viewer's left and the anterior aspect of the patient will be at the top of the image. Sagittal images will be presented with the apex of the prostate to the viewer's left and the rectum at the top of the image.

In real time the transducer is advanced to the level of the confluence of the vas deferens and seminal vesicles and manipulated into the plane which best depicts the symmetry of both seminal vesicles. This manuever should ensure that the transducer is accurately positioned axially to the long axis of the seminal vesicles and the prostate gland. It is important to take the time to arrive at this plane otherwise any conclusion regarding seminal vesicle or prostatic symmetry, or lack thereof, may be misleading. (Figure 1)

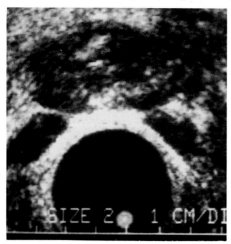

Figure 1. The transducer has been positioned parallel to the long axis of the seminal vesicles and prostate and nicely demonstrates the seminal vesicle-prostatic angles bilaterally.

Multiple imaging sweeps are performed from the seminal vesicles through the apex and selected sweeps are recorded on video tape. One can often obtain better images if the probe is hand held. However, the use of a mechnical stepping device to hold the transducer may be utilized. The use of frozen stepped images taken at 5mm increments is discouraged as one may step across a 5mm abnormality and never detect its presence.

It is important to understand the focal properties of the transducer element utilized so that the transducer may be positioned within the rectum with the focal zone encompasssing the area of interest. The system gain should be adjusted to present information from low level reflectors as well as strong prominent reflectors such as the glandular capsule. A grey scale assignment scheme should be used to accurately depict the intensity of the returning echoes in a linear fashion. Once a satisfactory grey scale assignment scheme has been found, one should avoid post-processing the image to make an equivocal finding look abnormal.

We feel that the examination should be performed in both the axial and sagittal projections. Although we do not have any objective data we would be uncomfortable with imaging in just the sagittal plane. However, we believe that "screening" could be performed with only an axial device.

Advantages of axial imaging include the following:

   - assessment of glandular left-right symmetry

   - ability to compare peripheral zone echotexture of both left and right sides simultaneously

   - assessment of the anterior lateral

region of the peripheral zone

— ability to readily appreciate the vessels of the neurovascular bundles entering the peripheral zone

— ability to better assess the extraglandular spread of neoplasm

— with a needle guide system, to perform an orthogonal biopsy of suspicious areas

— with a stepping device, to readily calculate glandular volume

— with an implantation template, to ultrasonically implant radioactive sources into the gland. (Figures 2-4)

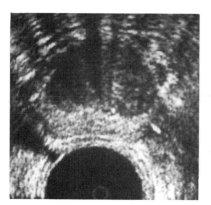

Figure 2.

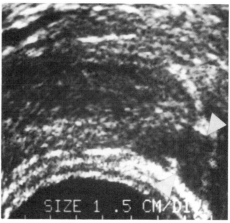

Figure 3.

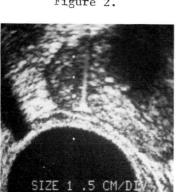

Figure 4.

Figure 2. Axial image demonstrates glandular symmetry and allows comparison of echotexture of both sides of the peripheral zone tissue.

Figure 3. Note the large blood vessel entering the peripheral zone tissue on the left side (arrowheads). Axial image near gland apex.

Figure 4. A needle has been placed into a suspicious area in the right peripheral zone in an orthogonal fashion using a biopsy guide. Note the large echo from the needle tip and the reverberation artifact.

Advantages of sagittal imaging include the following:

— confirmation of the presence of a small lesion

— superior evaluation of the apex and base of the gland

— accurately measure the cephalocaudad extent of a lesion

— to confirm the relationship of the tip of a biopsy needle to an abnormality

— evaluate disease processes involving the ejaculatory ductal systems. (Figures 5-8)

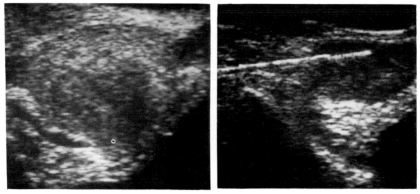

Figure 5.

Figure 6.

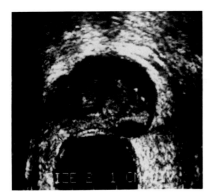

Figure 7.

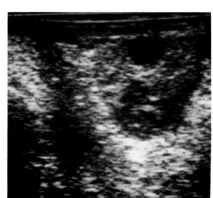

Figure 8.

Figure 5. Midline sagittal image which clearly demonstrates the apex and base of the gland.

Figure 6. Sagittal image of a transperineal co-axial biopsy with the tip of a 19 guage histology needle seen within the hypoechoic neoplasm; the tip of the 14 guage needle lies just within the capsule of the prostate gland.

Figure 7. Axial image demonstrates an abnormal hypoechoic area in the peripheral zone on the left side.

Figure 8. Sagittal image of the same patient as in Figure 7 demonstrating the cephalocaudad extent of the abnormal area. Pathological diagnosis: granulomatous prostatitis.

Some of the artifacts that may result in a suboptimal examination include excessive gas within the rectum, small residual particles of fecal material which will cause an acoustic shadow across the peripheral zone, and reverberation artifacts from the condom or prostate capsule. Figures 9-10.

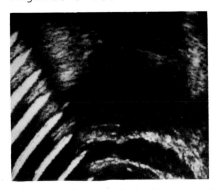 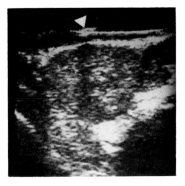

Figure 9. Multiple parallel reverberation artifacts from gas between the water filled condom and the rectal wall obscure the right side of this axial scan.

Figure 10. Small particles of fecal material

(arrowhead) absorbs some of the ultrasonic energy
and casts a shadow across this sagittal image of
the prostate gland.

By taking the time to understand the physics
of ultrasound and the functions of the various
controls on the scanning device used one can
greatly improve the quality of the examination of
the prostate gland.

The Use of Transrectal Ultrasound in the Diagnosis and
Management of Prostate Cancer, pages 57–71
© 1987 Alan R. Liss, Inc.

DIAGNOSTIC CONSIDERATIONS IN TRANSRECTAL ULTRASONIC
IMAGING OF THE PROSTATE GLAND

Glen H. Kumasaka, M.D.
Department of Radiology, St. Joseph
Mercy Hospital, Ann Arbor, MI 48106

Transrectal ultrasonic imaging of the prostate
gland can depict the major divisions and structures
of this small and complex organ. Utilizing the
model and concept of McNeal, we divide the organ
into an anterior component consisting of the
urethra and its musculostromal complex and a
posterior component comprising the glandular tissue
and ejaculatory apparatus. (McNeal, 1968) The
centrally placed urethra and the surgical capsule
demarcate the plane between the two
compartments.(Figure 1)

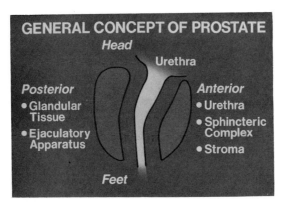

Figure 1. McNeal's conceptual model of the Prostate

The urethra is divided into two equal segments
by the angle which also locates the proximal end of
the ridged verumontanum. Into the distal urethral
segment empty the ducts of the prostatic gland and

the ejaculatory duct (EJ). Because of this
relationship with the glandular function, McNeal
terms this segment the prostatic urethra and the
proximal segment the pre-prostatic urethra. It is
in the region of the preprostatic urethra that the
benign hypertrophic process (BPH) develops.(McNeal,
1972) (Figure 2)

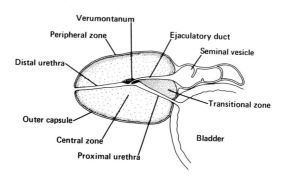

Figure 2. Graphic representation of the prostate
in sagittal projection. The distal urethra is
termed the prostatic urethra. The proximal urethra
is termed the pre-prostatic urethra.

McNeal, in his classic studies of the
prostate, has demonstrated that the hypertrophic
process of the central elements develops from two
distinct sites and tissues of origin. (McNeal,
1978) The tissue enlargement develops from stromal
tissue surrounding the pre-prostatic urethra. The
hypertrophic stroma apparently can then induce the
adjacent smooth muscle sheath of the internal
sphincter and the vestigial glands that are
embedded in the muscle to also hypertrophy. The
direction of this growth is towards the base of the
bladder. (Figures 3,4)

The major enlargement of the central gland
(CG) originates from the glandular tissue located
about the distal end of the pre-prostatic urethra.

This tissue, termed the transitional zone (TZ), is histologically separable from the parenchymal tissue (the peripheral zone, PZ) of the posterior zone. Like the peri-urethral process, the hypertrophic changes involve all three tissues consisting of gland, muscle and stroma. The direction of growth is anterior and lateral to the urethra.

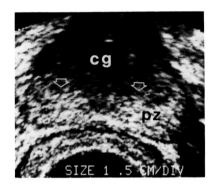 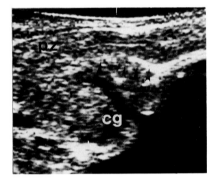

Figure 3. Normal axial view of the prostate:central gland (CG), peripheral zone (PZ), surgical capsule (arrowheads)
Figure 4. Normal sagittal view of the prostate.

The centrifugal out-growth of the central gland (CG) compresses the peripheral aspects of the inner gland to form a pseudo-capsule which is commonly termed the surgical capsule (SC). The parenchymal glandular tissue, the peripheral zone (PZ), of the prostate lies posterolateral to this margin and is identifiable as a tissue layer sandwiched between the surgical capsule and the true glandular capsule.

Finally, the paired diverging structures at the posterior base of the gland are the seminal vesicle (SV) with their closely associated vas deferens. (Figure 5)

ULTRASONIC CORRELATIONS:

Our standard ultrasonic images are recorded in axial and sagittal planes.

The fine glandular and ductal tissues of the peripheral zone lie within the posterior compartment, and present a homogeneous ultrasonic pattern. This is the baseline isoechogenicity to which other areas are compared. (Figure 6) Cancer, for example, appears as a dark, hypoechoic area within this homogeneous background.

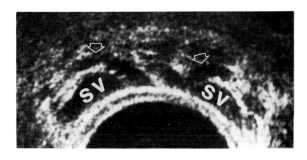

Figure 5. Axial view of seminal vesicles (SV) and vas deferens (arrowheads).

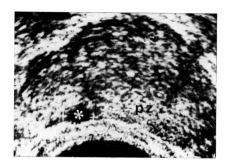

Figure 6. Cancer (*) in the peripheral zone (PZ).

The line of increased echo reflection from the prostatic capsule defines the posterior margin of the gland.

The ultrasonic key to evaluation of the prostate is the urethra and its central angle, which in the mid-sagittal section is frequently marked by a bright hyperechoic focus. (Figure 7) This point is related to a calcific deposit at the confluence of various tissue planes — the proximal end of the verumontanum and the angle of the urethra. (Dahnert, et al., 1986) Using this point as a landmark, we can delineate the course of the proximal and distal segments by projecting lines from it to the base of the bladder and to the apex of the gland.

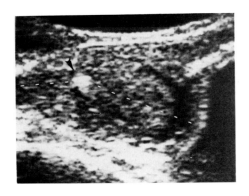

Figure 7. Calcific focus (arrow) at the midpoint of the urethra in sagittal section. The dotted line traces the proximal and distal urethra.

Lateral and cephalad to this central point is the surgical capsule which presents as a symmetrical, convex arc. This border is often accentuated by bright echogenic points which are related to corpora amylacea and calcifications deposited within atrophic glands along the surgical capsule. (Figure 8) Posterior to the surgical capsule is the homogeneous glandular tissue of the peripheral zone. Anteriorly, the central gland

(CG) makes up the zone of benign prostatic hypertrophy (BPH).

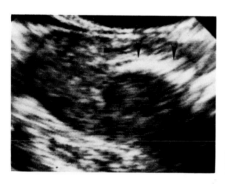 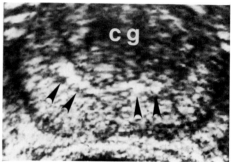

Figures 8a,b. A. Sagittal view showing deposition of calcifications along the surgical capsule. B. Axial view with calcifications and corpora amylacea, along the surgical capsule (arrowheads).

BENIGN PROSTATIC HYPERTROPHY (BPH):

The two distinct areas of enlargement and the three tissue elements of hypertrophy participate in varying proportions to produce unpredictable and varied ultrasonic patterns. (Figures 9 a,b,c) Hypoechoic, dark changes are related to compact glandular or muscular tissue. Mixed hypertrophic findings are usually complex glandular enlargement as well as interdigitating hypertrophic muscular, stromal and glandular tissues. Atrophic fluid filled glands result in tubular, punctate or confluent areas of hypoechoic texture. Calcifications are also scattered throughout.

However, as BPH progresses the general overall relationship of the gland remains relatively constant. (Figure 9d) The pressure of outward growth shapes the convex surgical capsule, accentuated by hyperechoic foci of corpora amylacea and calcifications. Postero-laterally to the central gland (CG) is the peripheral glandular parenchyma of the prostate.

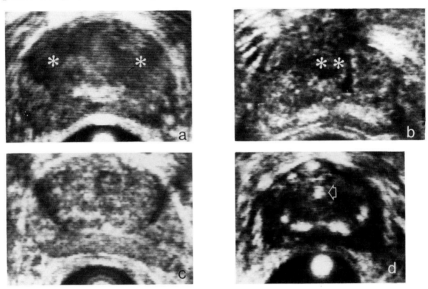

Figure 9 a,b,c. Axial views of the prostate demonstrating varied patterns (*) in the central gland resulting from intermixing of <u>differing</u> hypertrophic and atrophic structures. Figure 9 d. Overall relationship of the CG and PZ is still retained. Calcifications shown along the SC and about the urethra (arrow).

PROPOSAL FOR BPH STAGING:

With progressive growth of the central gland there is a continuum of changing contour in addition to the alteration in the inner pattern. We propose a four stage division based upon the contour of the gland, the CG/PZ ratio, the point of intersection of the SC with the gland contour, and lastly, the width of the PZ as it is compressed by the growing CG of the prostate.

In Stage I, the CG presents as a small oval in the anterocephalic aspect of the axial image with

the isoechoic PZ surrounding it.   The CG/PZ ratio
is much less than 1/1. (Figure 10)

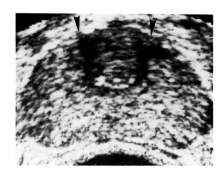

Figure 10.   Axial view, Stage I, small CG,
prominent PZ. Arrowheads delineate margin of the
SC.

     With progressive enlargement of the CG, the
central pattern expands anteriorly, laterally and
caudally. The criteria for Stage II involve the
lateral migration of the SC margin to the
anterolateral point of the prostatic outline and
the CG/PZ ratio approaches unity. (Figure 11a) The
PZ now cups the lateral and posterior aspects of
the CG.

     A variation of Stage II displays a pear shaped
contour which results when the enlargement process
involves more selectively the pre-prostatic periurethral tissues rather than the more usual
hypertrophy of the TZ. The former tissue enlarges
cephalad resulting in an anterior bulging of the CG
contour. (Figure 11b)

     In Stage III there is further increase in the
CG/PZ ratio (greater than one) and the SC juncture
now moves posteriorly along the lateral contour.
The PZ width continues to remain relatively full,
its AP measurement being one centimeter or more.
(Figure 12)

Stage IV specifically differs from Stage III in the notable thinning of the PZ width, which now is less than one centimeter. The CG/PZ ratio increases and there is further posterior migration of the SC margin. The volume of the CG now dominates the entire picture. (Figure 13)

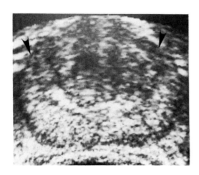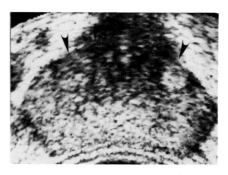

Figures 11a,b. A. Stage II, enlarging CG with SC margin (arrow) migrating laterally, CG/PZ ratio approches unity. B. Stage II variant, SC margin (arrow) moves laterally.

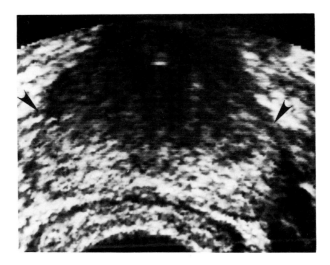

Figure 12. Stage III, further CG enlargement with CG/PZ ratio greater than unity — PZ width equal to 1 cm.

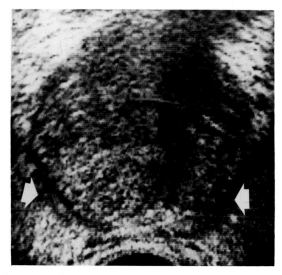

Figure 13. Axial view of Stage IV, CG/PZ ratio much greater than unity, PZ (arrow) width less than 1 cm.

Since there is no direct correlation of the hypertrophied CG with obstructive symptoms, we postulate that the thinning of the PZ width can be an indicator of the anatomical contribution to voiding dysfunction. In the absence of advanced Stage III and IV changes, neuromuscular dysfunction is probably the major significant determinant of obstructive symptoms.

PZ CONSIDERATIONS:

Within the narrow isoechoic band that makes up the peripheral zone are hypoechoic and hyperechoic changes. One often encounters hyperechoic findings which entend from the central area to the peripheral zone. (Figures 14a,b) These are dystrophic calcifications secondary to previous inflammations or infarctions. This is a benign finding to which no further attention need be paid.

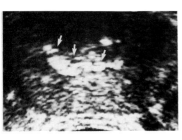 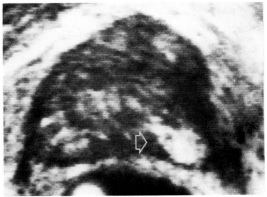

Figures 14a, b. A.Calcifications in CG along SC (arrows). B. Calcifications (arrow) in the PZ.

Since carcinoma presents as a dark region, the prime differential consideration is to evaluate hypoechoic changes in this zone. (Figure 15) There are miscellaneous conditions whose images are identical to carcinoma. Those hypoechoic entities that one may encounter included the following structures and inflammatory processes:

> Granulomatous Prostatitis (Figure 16)
> Atypical Glandular Hyperplasia
> Atrophic and Dysplastic Glands
> Leiomyomatous Hyperplasia
> Dilated ducts and cysts
> Neurovascular Bundles
> Blood Vessels and Vascular Lakes
> Muscle around the Ejaculatory Ducts
> The Muscular External Sphincter

At present biopsy is the only means to determine the underlying pathology.

The muscular sheath surrounding the ejaculatory duct (EJ) presents in sagittal projection as a hypoechoic arc which extends from the seminal vesicles to the verumontanum. (Figure 17) In the axial plane, it will present as a hypoechoic dot in the basal aspect of the PZ. Abnormally distended SV and ejaculatory ducts caused by an obstructing stone or scarring at the

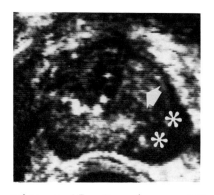 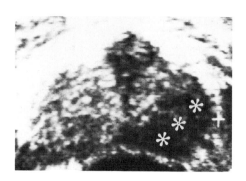

Figure 15. Carcinoma (*) along the left side of the PZ with invasion into the CG (arrow).
Figure 16. Prostatitis in the left side of the PZ (*).

verumontanum are also encountered. An occasional cyst-like dilatation of the proximal EJ occurs at the cephalic end of the posterior prostate. (Figures 18a,b) It seems to arise at the juncture of the SV and vas deferens and may represent a bulging at a weakened area. The PZ is moderately narrow at the point of insertion of the EJ and conceivably may narrow the ductal lumen.

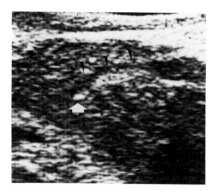

Figure 17. Sagittal view with normal configuration of ejaculatory duct (arrowheads) and verumontanum (white arrow).

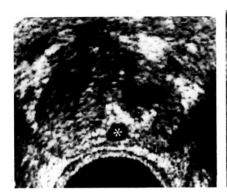
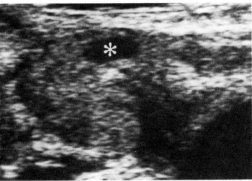

Figure 18a,b.   A. Ejaculatory duct cyst (*) shown in axial projection. B. EJ cyst in sagittal view.

Neurovascular bundles in the subcapsular region can closely mimic a small carcinoma on a single isolated image. (Figure 19) Careful probe movement in real time can follow this suspicious area out through the capsule and into the

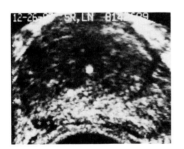
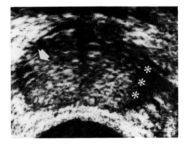

Figure 19.   Neurovascular bundle (*).
Figure 20.   Vascular "blush" along dependent (left) side of prostate gland, vessels on right side (arrow).

extraglandular vascular channels. A more trouble- some finding is a hypoechoic "blush" seen on the left side along the mid portion of the PZ. (Figure 20) This frequent finding on the left side is secondary to the left lateral decubitous position of the patient. The darkened region is the result of capillary congestion and increased fluid content on the dependent side.

An equally bothersome hypoechoic pattern is often present at the apex of the gland in the sagittal projection. When biopsied one obtains striated muscular tissue from the external sphincter. The dark capping can be altered into a linear pattern when the patient is asked to constrict the muscles of the pelvic floor. This maneuver has been incorporated as a routine part of our examination. (Figures 21a,b)

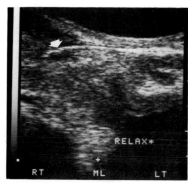 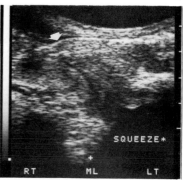

Figures 21a,b. A. Sagittal view shows hypoechoic striated muscle tissue at the gland apex. B. Suspicious hypoechoic area disappears when muscles of the pelvic floor are contracted.

SEMINAL VESICLE (SV):

The SV presents a paired, wing-like hypoechoic structure which radiates laterally from the postero-caphalic aspect of the base of the prostate. It appears as a symmetrical, slightly irregularly textured cylinder in the decompressed state. When engorged with seminal fluid the organs can double in overall cross section with tortuous, fluid-filled tubules. On occasion one can visualize peristaltic activity within the seminal vesicles secondary to stimulation of the nerves within the capsule of the prostate.

CONCLUSION:

We are now able to ultrasonically image with accuracy the various structures of the prostate gland. McNeal's concept of the benign anterior process of BPH and the varing condition (including carcinoma) in the posterior zone can be translated into meaningful patterns.

A proposed staging of BPH and a brief description of the ejaculatory apparatus and seminal vesicles are presented.

REFERENCES

Dähnert, WR, Hamper, UM, Walsh, PC, Eggleston, JC, Walsh PC, Sanders, RC (1986). Prostatic Evaluation by Transrectal Sonography with Histopathologic Correlation: The Echopenic Appearance of Early Carcinoma. Radiology 158:1:97-102.

McNeal, JE (1968). Regional Morphology of the Prostate. Am J Clin Path 49:369.

McNeal, JE (1972). The Prostate and Prostatic Urethra: A Morphologic Synthesis. J Urol 107: 1008.

McNeal, JE (1978). Origin and Evolution of Benign Prostatic Enlargement. Invest Urolo 15: 340.

The Use of Transrectal Ultrasound in the Diagnosis and
Management of Prostate Cancer, pages 73–109
© 1987 Alan R. Liss, Inc.

TRANSRECTAL ULTRASOUND IN THE DIAGNOSIS, STAGING, GUIDED
NEEDLE BIOPSY, AND SCREENING FOR PROSTATE CANCER

Fred Lee, M.D.

Department of Radiology, St. Joseph Mercy
Hospital, P.O. Box 995 Ann Arbor, Michigan
48106

INTRODUCTION

Prostate cancer is the second most common malignancy
and the third most common cause of death due to cancer in
men (Cancer Statistics, 1985). An autopsy series of men
over 50 years of age who died of other causes demonstrated
that about 30% had unsuspected cancer of the prostate
(Franks, 1954). The occurrence of prostate cancer in
tissue removed at transurethral resection is approximately
10% for the 50-60 age group, increasing with each subsequent
decade (Sheldon et al, 1980).

Once a carcinoma of the prostate enlarges beyond a
critical size, variously described as 1.0-1.5 cm in diameter,
the potential for a cure is much diminished. Long term
survival of patients following radical prostatectomy show
maximal longevity with cancers up to 1.0 cm, slight decreasing
survival with lesions up to 1.5 cm and progressive decrease
in survival with lesions over 1.5 cm in size. Therefore,
to be clinically useful, a diagnostic method must consistently
detect the cancer before it reaches 1.0 to 1.5 cm in diameter
(McNeal, 1969; Scott, 1969; Stamey, 1983; Culp, Meyer, 1973).

Various imaging modalities have been used in an attempt
to detect cancer of the prostate gland. At present,
computed tomography and magnetic resonance imaging are not
capable of reliably identifying small cancers confined to
the prostate gland (Emory et al, 1983; Rickards et al, 1983;
Golimbu M et al, 1981; Bryan et al 1983; Ling et al, 1986).
Of the various ultrasound methods used to image the prostate,

transrectal scanning best demonstrates normal and pathologic changes (Rifkin et al, 1983). We and others have shown that transrectal ultrasound (TRUS) can diagnose and detect the early stages of prostate cancer (Lee et al, 1986; Dahnert et al 1986). Its previously low reported specificity has prevented widespread acceptance (Rifkin et al, 1983; Fritzsche et al, 1983).

In the following chapter, our studies demonstrate TRUS to be the diagnostic imaging tool of choice in the study of prostate cancer. We intend to:

1. Characterize the ultrasound criteria for prostate cancer and to clarify the confusing echo-patterns described for it in the recent literature (Rifkin et al, 1983; Fritzsche et al, 1983, Watanabe et al, 1975; Resnick et al, 1978; Peeling et al, 1979; Rifkin et al, 1986).

2. Use these diagnostic criteria to formulate our ultrasound staging system for prostate cancer. It is a modification of Whitmore's clinical staging system and is based primarily on tumor size (Whitmore, 1956; Schmidt, 1985).

3. Describe a new biplane ultrasound guided biopsy technique in order to more easily sample small suspicious areas of the prostate. Since the size of the cancer and its potential for capsular penetration are closely linked, it is important that these areas be biopsied at an early stage in hopes of having a potential cure (Lee et al, Accepted for Publication in Radiology).

4. Show its potential use in an early detection program comparing TRUS with the digital rectal examination (DRE).

MATERIALS AND METHODS

Axial and sagittal scans were obtained in all studies using a Bruel & Kjaer (B & K) Model 1846 scanner with 5.5 and 7.0 MHz transducers and an Aloka 256 scanner with a

5.0 MHz transducer. All studies were recorded on multi-format film and 3/4" videotape.

Our ultrasound criteria for prostate cancer is an anechoic/hypoechoic lesion originating in the peripheral zone (PZ) of the gland. All suspicious lesions were measured in three dimensions (length/width/height) and the average diameter and cubic volume computed. These lesions were ultrasonically staged using our modification of Whitmore's clinical system (Fig. 1).

The anatomic nomenclature used in this paper is a modification of the work of McNeal (McNeal, 1968; McNeal, 1983). We divide the gland into an outer peripheral zone and an inner central gland. The peripheral zone tissue is covered on its outer aspect by the prostatic capsule. The peripheral zone occupies mainly the posterior, lateral and apical aspects of the gland. The tissues of the central zone, the transition zone, and the anterior fibromuscular stroma compose the central gland. At this time, the central gland areas cannot be individually distinguished with ultrasound. The central gland tissue is enclosed along its apical, posterior and lateral aspects by an echogenic interface which corresponds to the "surgical capsule".

We have found that the normal peripheral zone is homogenous in appearance and has an echogenicity in our laboratory which we consider isoechoic. The ultrasound appearance of the remainder of the gland and any abnormalities, whether benign or malignant, are compared to this standard.

DIAGNOSIS AND STAGING

Over a fourteen month period, 1343 patients were examined with transrectal ultrasound. The majority of these patients presented with palpable abnormalities or obstructive symptoms. They ranged in age from 20 to 96 with a mean age of 60.

Twenty-nine whole prostates obtained at autopsy or by radical prostatectomy were examined. Thirteen out of 18 cancers in this series were from our own clinical study. Two others were found in autopsy specimens and three

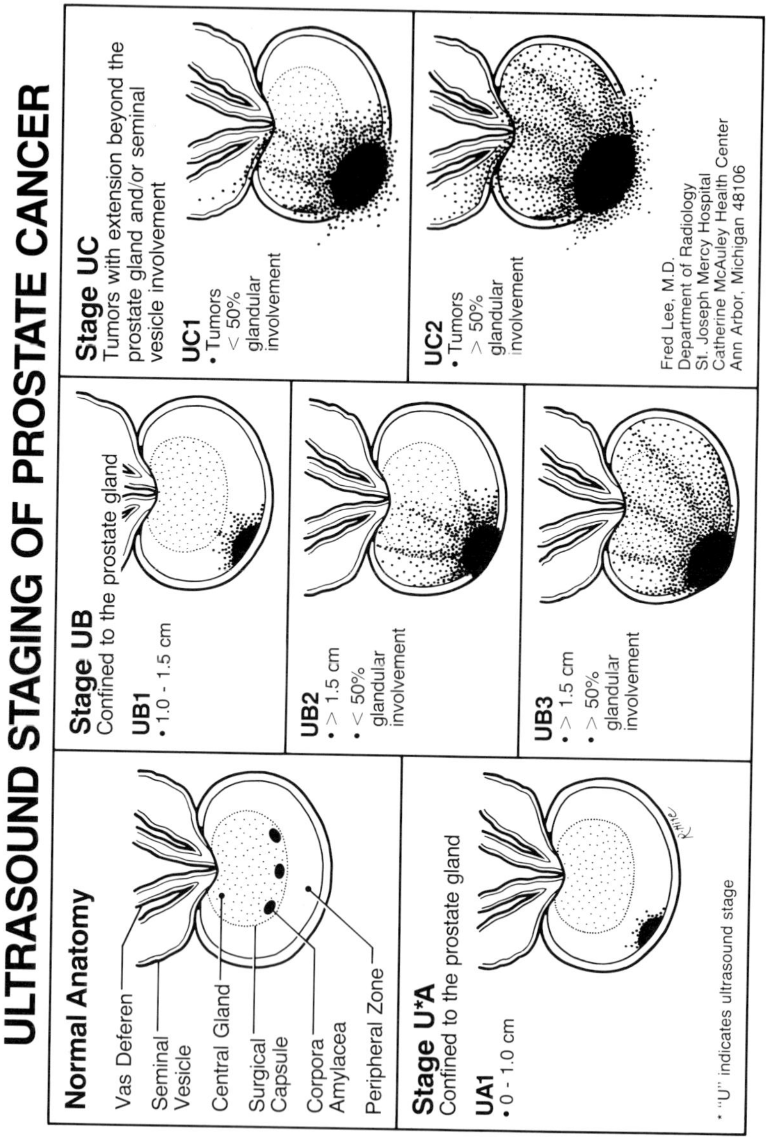

ULTRASOUND STAGING OF PROSTATE CANCER

Normal Anatomy

- Vas Deferen
- Seminal Vesicle
- Central Gland
- Surgical Capsule
- Corpora Amylacea
- Peripheral Zone

Stage U*A
Confined to the prostate gland

UA1
- 0 - 1.0 cm

Stage UB
Confined to the prostate gland

UB1
- 1.0 - 1.5 cm

UB2
- > 1.5 cm
- < 50% glandular involvement

UB3
- > 1.5 cm
- > 50% glandular involvement

Stage UC
Tumors with extension beyond the prostate gland and/or seminal vesicle involvement

UC1
- Tumors < 50% glandular involvement

UC2
- Tumors > 50% glandular involvement

Fred Lee, M.D.
Department of Radiology
St. Joseph Mercy Hospital
Catherine McAuley Health Center
Ann Arbor, Michigan 48106

* "U" indicates ultrasound stage

FIGURE 1

cancerous specimens were from another institution. These prostates were scanned in a water bath with images obtained at 5 mm intervals in axial and sagittal planes. The glands were then fixed in formalin, processed, sectioned for whole mount study and stained with hematoxylin and eosin. The plane of section chosen for whole mount preparation was that corresponding to the ultrasound projection that best demonstrated any abnormality.

BIPLANE ULTRASOUND GUIDED BIOPSY TECHNIQUE

In a six month period, eighty patients (83 biopsies) underwent 22 gauge cytologic [1] aspiration and 14 gauge histologic [2] biopsies of suspicious lesions seen on TRUS. Twenty-one of these patients also had 19 gauge fine needle aspiration histology. The DRE of the patient prior to biopsy showed that 56% had a discrete nodule, 24% a suspicious abnormality and 20% no abnormality.

A baseline blood pressure and pulse are obtained. The patient should have no bleeding tendency and not be on anticoagulants. No premedications were given.

The following is the biopsy procedure that we utilized (Fig. 2):

1. The patient is placed in a left lateral decubitus position, semi-fetal, for both scanning and biopsying.

2. Local anesthesia is given transperineally using 10-15 cc's of 1% Xylocaine through a 22 gauge needle (15 cm length). The appropriate notch for needle insertion is selected by matching the puncture guide overlay as it is projected over the lesion in real-time using the axial probe. A modified needle biopsy guide for the B & K axial probe is used to direct the placement of the local anesthesia.

3. A 14 gauge needle (4") is advanced two to three inches into the perineum but not into the prostate. Its inner trocar is then removed.

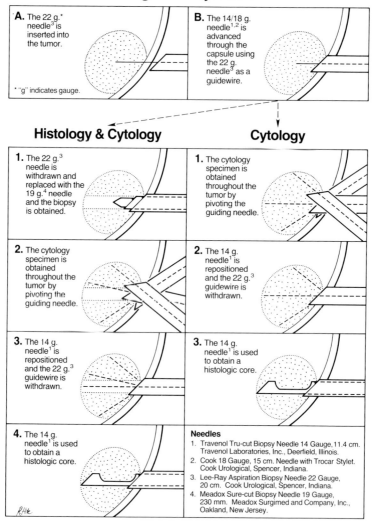

BIOPSY TECHNIQUES
Sagittal Projection

A. The 22 g.* needle[3] is inserted into the tumor.

* "g" indicates gauge.

B. The 14/18 g. needle[1,2] is advanced through the capsule using the 22 g. needle[3] as a guidewire.

Histology & Cytology

1. The 22 g.[3] needle is withdrawn and replaced with the 19 g.[4] needle and the biopsy is obtained.

2. The cytology specimen is obtained throughout the tumor by pivoting the guiding needle.

3. The 14 g. needle[1] is repositioned and the 22 g.[3] guidewire is withdrawn.

4. The 14 g. needle[1] is used to obtain a histologic core.

Cytology

1. The cytology specimen is obtained throughout the tumor by pivoting the guiding needle.

2. The 14 g. needle[1] is repositioned and the 22 g.[3] guidewire is withdrawn.

3. The 14 g. needle[1] is used to obtain a histologic core.

Needles
1. Travenol Tru-cut Biopsy Needle 14 Gauge, 11.4 cm. Travenol Laboratories, Inc., Deerfield, Illinois.
2. Cook 18 Gauge, 15 cm. Needle with Trocar Stylet. Cook Urological, Spencer, Indiana.
3. Lee-Ray Aspiration Biopsy Needle 22 Gauge, 20 cm. Cook Urological, Spencer, Indiana.
4. Meadox Sure-cut Biopsy Needle 19 Gauge, 230 mm. Meadox Surgimed and Company, Inc., Oakland, New Jersey.

FIGURE 2

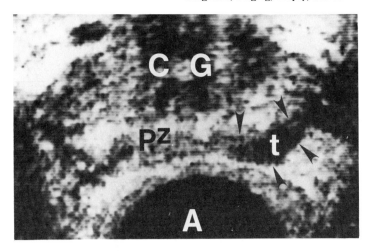

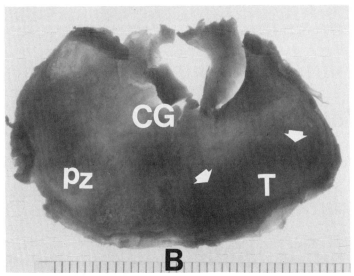

FIGURE 3 (A,B):   STAGE UB1, palpable cancer, Gleason grade 5
                  capsular invasion level 2.
                  A, B show tumor (T) (arrowheads) involving
                  the left peripheral zone (PZ).

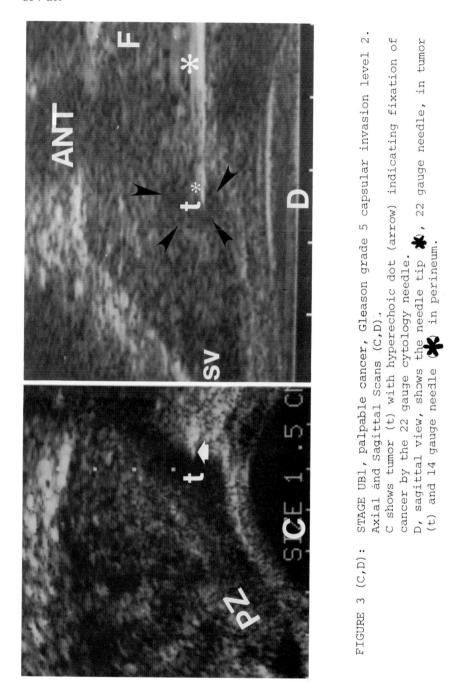

FIGURE 3 (C,D): STAGE UB1, palpable cancer, Gleason grade 5 capsular invasion level 2.
Axial and Sagittal Scans (C,D).
C shows tumor (t) with hyperechoic dot (arrow) indicating fixation of
cancer by the 22 gauge cytology needle.
D, sagittal view, shows the needle tip ✱, 22 gauge needle, in tumor
(t) and 14 gauge needle ✿ in perineum.

4. The 22 gauge cytology needle is advanced
    into the 14 gauge needle's outer sheath and
    into the suspicious lesion under ultrasound
    guidance. This appears as a focal hyperechoic
    dot with a typical metallic comet tail shadow
    (Fig. 3).

    To achieve definitive placement of the
    22 gauge needle (especially for small lesions
    less than 1.0 cm) the 14 gauge needle is
    removed from the B & K needle guide and the
    22 gauge needle is guided by manual manip-
    ulation to the anechoic-hypoechoic tumor.

    Milling of the guiding grooves to produce
    vertical side walls was necessary to allow
    removal of the 14 gauge needle from the
    needle guide of the axial probe.

5. The axial probe is removed and the sagittal
    probe inserted. The needle can be visualized
    throughout its length and its tip can now
    be ascertained to be in the lesion.

6. The tip of the 14 gauge needle is advanced
    up to caudal edge of the lesion using the
    22 gauge as a guidewire.

7. A 10 cc plastic syringe for aspiration is
    attached to the 22 gauge cytologic needle.
    Maintaining constant negative pressure rapid
    in and out needle tip movements are made
    throughout various areas of the lesion.

    The negative pressure is released with the
    tip of the 22 gauge needle in the lesion.

8. The 22 gauge needle is removed and cytological
    smears are made. The needle's central stylet
    is replaced and any remaining tissue is
    extruded into normal saline to make a cell
    block.

9. The central stylet of the 14 gauge needle is
    replaced and tissue cores are obtained of the
    lesion.

Blood pressure and pulse are again obtained
and the patient is discharged when stable.
No special instructions are given. Anti-
biotics are not usually prescribed.

In the last 21 cases, we also used a 19 gauge aspiration
histology needle for the initial biopsy beginning after step
6. The tip of the 19 gauge needle is placed in the lesion
and negative pressure is then applied. The needle is
rapidly advanced a number of times into the lesion and then
rotated to dislodge an impacted tissue core. The core is
expelled onto sterile filter paper in a linear fashion as
the suction is released. It is stained with eosin and
placed with the paper into formalin. The 22 gauge needle
is then used after the 19 gauge to obtain cytology.

When the 14 gauge needle is not used, it is replaced
by an 18 gauge guiding needle with trocar, step 3, [4]
through which the 22 and 19 gauge needles can easily pass.
This 18 gauge needle is used only as a stabilizing guide
for the thin needles.

EARLY DETECTION PROGRAM COMPARING TRUS VERSUS DIGITAL
RECTAL EXAMINATION

Three hundred eighty-eight patients were examined from
June 1985 through January 1986. Subjects were self-referred,
at least 60 years of age and had no history of prostate
surgery. Subjects were independently studied by TRUS and
DRE (in a blind fashion).

If either the radiologist or urologist detected an
abnormality and recommended a biopsy, it was then performed
under local anesthesia in the out-patient department.

[1]   Lee-Ray Aspiration Biopsy Needle 22 Gauge,
        20 cm. Cook Urological, Spencer, Indiana.
[2]   Travenol Tru-Cut Biopsy Needle 14 Gauge,
        11.4 cm. Travenol Laboratories, Inc.,
        Dearfield, Illinois.
[3]   Meadox Sure-Cut Biopsy Needle 19 Gauge, 230 mm.
        Meadox Surgimed and Company, Inc., Oakland,
        New Jersey.
[4]   Cook 18 Gauge, 15 cm Needle with Trocar Stylet.
      Cook Urological, Spencer, Indiana.

RESULTS

Diagnosis and Staging

One hundred and eighteen lesions were proven to be adenocarcinoma. The appearance of all of these were consistent with our ultrasound criteria for cancer. These criteria are a hypoechoic lesion which appears to originate within the peripheral zone tissue (Lee et al, 1985). We were able to appreciate an anechoic focus within these hypoechoic cancers when imaged at 7.0 MHz. Because of this finding, our current criteria for a small cancer of the prostate is an anechoic or hypoechoic focus originating in the peripheral zone. Nine additional cases were found to be atypical glandular hyperplasia (Kastendieck et al, 1976; Helpap, 1980). The mean age for patients with cancer was 70, ranging from 53 to 90 years of age. The 118 cancers and 9 atypical glandular hyperplasias were proven by the following means: 89 by ultrasound guided transperineal biopsies, twenty-two by finger guided biopsies, and thirteen by tissue obtained from transurethral resection. In addition, three cases presented with distant metastases.

One case in this series of 118 cancers was a biopsy proven recurrence following total prostatectomy with development of a mass in the region of the prostatic bed. The recurrent cancer was hypoechoic in appearance and histologically well differentiated.

Results of staging according to our modification of the Whitmore's clinical staging system and histologic grading are contained in table 1.

One hundred and seventeen cancers were grouped according to size. Eleven cancers were less than 1.0 cm in average diameter, 19 were from 1.0 to 1.5 cm in average diameter, 44 were larger than 1.5 cm with up to 50% involvement of the gland, and 13 involved more than 50% of the gland. Twenty-eight cancers presented with extra-capsular spread and of these, eight involved the seminal vesicles. Two cancers had seminal vesicle involvement without extra-capsular extension. The 118th case, a local recurrence after total prostatectomy, was not assigned a size. The larger tumors tended to be less well differentiated and were associated with greater capsular involvement and/or penetration (Table 1).

The eighteen whole mount specimens with cancer were grouped according to size and Gleason grade (Table 2). Four cancers were less than 1.0 cm in average diameter. Two cancers, 3.0 and 4.0 mm in average diameter, with a Gleason grade of 2 were not detected by ultrasound. These were imaged with 5.0 and 5.5 MHz transducers. The other two cancers, less than 1.0 cm in diameter, were easily seen at 7.0 MHz and were Gleason grade 4 (Fig. 4). No extra-capsular spread was detected. Eight cancers greater than 1.0 cm but less than 1.5 cm in average diameter were found, four of which were Gleason grades of 5 or less with no evident capsular penetration (Fig. 5,6). The four remaining specimens had microscopic extra-prostatic spread and Gleason grades all above 5 (Fig. 7). Six cancers greater than 1.5 cm in average size were found. One specimen, containing a cancer greater than 1.5 cm in average diameter and Gleason grade of 4, had in addition a second cancer 0.5 cm in diameter present on the contra-lateral side which was not detected using 5.0 and 5.5 MHz transducers (Fig.8). All but one had extra-prostatic microscopic spread (Fig. 9). One specimen showed tumor enveloping the aditus of the seminal vesicle producing dilatation of the seminal vesicle duct and enlargement of the involved seminal vesicle (Fig. 10). The Gleason grade of these six cancers ranged from 4 to 9.

RESULTS OF THE FINE NEEDLE CYTOLOGY AND HISTOLOGY VERSUS LARGE CORE BIOPSY

Table 3 cross-categorizes the diagnostic results of the 22 gauge cytology and 14 gauge histology needles. Five lesions diagnosed as benign by histology were definitive for cancer by cytology. Four of these five lesions were confirmed cancers on additional 19 gauge or finger guided biopsies and one remained benign on re-biopsy. All cytology read as suspicious for malignancy was proven to be cancer by histology, or in one case by re-biopsy. On the other hand, one benign cytologic diagnosis had a histologic finding of cancer. Eleven (13%) of the cytologic studies were inadequate for diagnosis. Six of these eleven (55%) were diagnosed as cancer by histology. Three of the five patients with diagnoses of atypical glandular hyperplasia had received radiation therapy for previously diagnosed prostate cancer.

TABLE 1

DEGREE OF HISTOLOGIC DIFFERENTIATION VS.
ULTRASOUND STAGING (TUMOR SIZE)

	UA	UB1	UB2	UB3	UC1	UC2
Age	68.2	68.0	68.8	68.8	70.6	73.0
HISTOLOGY:						
Well	11 (100%)	14 (74%)	21 (48%)	3 (25%)	1 (17%)	4 (21%)
Well to Moderate		1 (5%)	3 (7%)	2 (17%)	1 (17%)	1 (5%)
Moderate		1 (5%)	15 (34%)	6 (50%)	2 (33%)	2 (10%)
Moderate to Poor		2 (11%)	4 (9%)	1 (8%)	1 (17%)	4 (21%)
Undifferentiated		1 (5%)	1 (2%)		1 (17%)	8 (42%)
TOTAL:	11	19	44	12	6	19
No Grade, Known CA &/or Metastatic Disease (6)				1	2	3
Local Recurrence 1	1					
Total CA (118)	12	19	44	13	8	22
Atypical Hyperplasia (9)	7	2				

GRAND TOTAL: 127 (Cancer [118] and Atypical Hyperplasia [9])

TABLE 2

GLEASON GRADE VS. TUMOR SIZE IN CENTIMETERS
WHOLE MOUNT SERIES
(N = 18)

SIZE (cm)	UA 0.0-1.0	UB1 1.0-1.5	UB2 > 1.5 (< 50%)	UB3 > 1.5 (> 50%)	UC1	UC2
GLEASON GRADE:						
2	2 (−)	1 (−)				
3		1 (−)				
4	2 (−)	2 (−)	1 (+)			
5		1 (−)	1 (+)			
6						
7		1 (+)	1 (+)	1 (−)	1 (+)	
8		2 (+)				
9						1 (+)
10						
TOTAL: 18	4	8	3	1	1	1

(+) = Capsular Penetration

TABLE 3

ULTRASOUND GUIDED TRANSPERINEAL BIOPSIES
22g. Cytology vs. 14 g. Histology *

Cytology		Histology				
		Cancer	Atypical	Benign	Prostatitis	Insufficient
Cancer	38	33	0	5	0	0
Suspicious	6	5	0	0	0	1
Atypical	2	0	2	0	0	0
Benign	25	1	3	18	1	2
Prostatitis	1	0	0	0	1	0
Insufficient	11	6	0	5	0	0
TOTAL	83	45	5	28	2	3
				83		

	CYTOLOGY	HISTOLOGY
CANCER	53% (38/72)	58% (46/80)
CA + SUSPICIOUS	61% (44/72)	58% (46/80)
COMBINED CYTOLOGY & HISTOLOGY	61% (51/83)	

*Comparisons are for those studies with sufficient tissue for pathologic diagnosis.

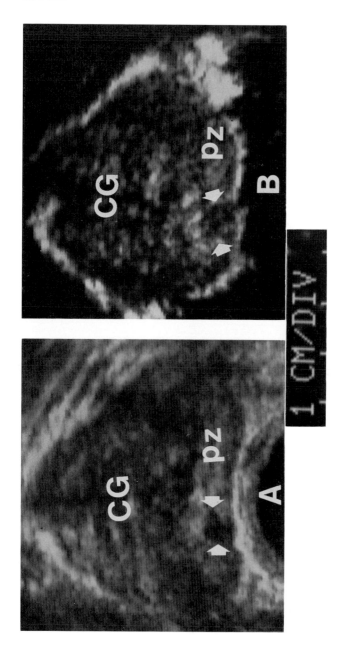

FIGURE 4 (A,B):   STAGE UA, non-palpable cancer, Gleason grade 2+2
                  capsular invasion level 2.
                  Axial scans in vivo (A) and in vitro (B) scans show
                  tumor T (arrows) in peripheral zone (PZ).

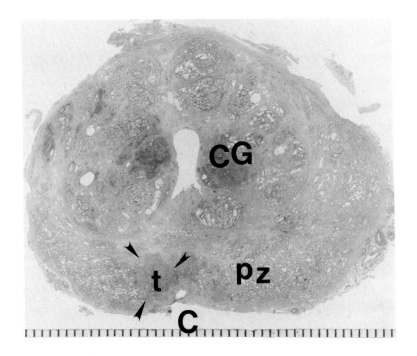

FIGURE 4 (C):   STAGE UA, non-palpable cancer, Gleason
                grade 2+2 capsular invasion level 2.
                C shows tumor t (arrowheads).

    When biopsies with sufficient tissue are considered,
the positive biopsy results of the two methods is similar:
Sixty-one percent (44/72) of the samples were diagnosed as
cancer or suspicious for cancer by cytology and 58% (46/80)
by histology. Combining the positive diagnoses for cytology
and/or histology, gives an overall positive biopsy rate of
61% (51/83) (Table 3). The positive biopsy yield of cytology
versus histology were essentially equal for all ultrasound
stages (Fig. 11). Positive biopsies were obtained in 34%
of stage UA, 56% of stage UB1 lesions and 96% of lesions
stage UB2 and greater (Fig. 12).

    The DRE results by ultrasound stage for the 49 patients
with biopsy proven cancer are: Sixty-seven percent (6/9) of
the patients with stage UA and 50% (7/14) with stage UB1

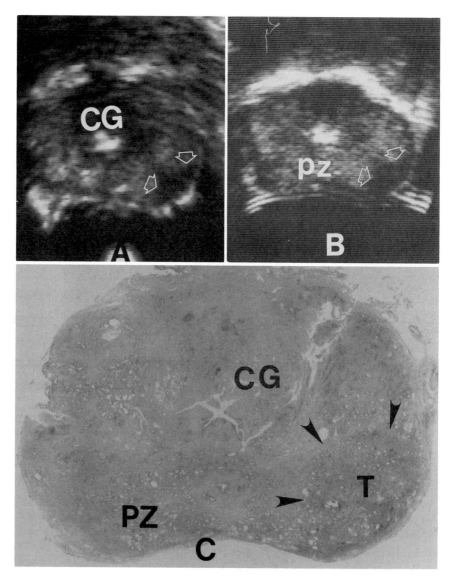

FIGURE 5 (A,B,C):   STAGE UB1, palpable cancer, Gleason
grade 2+2 capsular invasion level 1.
Axial scans (A,B) show tumor (arrows)
and axial (C) whole mount section shows
tumor T (arrowheads). CG = central gland
PZ = peripheral zone.

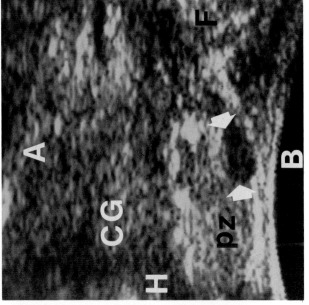

FIGURE 6 (A,B): STAGE UB1, non-palpable cancer, Gleason grade 2+2 capsular invasion level 2.
Axial scan (A) and sagittal scan (B) show tumor (arrows).
A = anterior, H = head, F = feet, CG = central gland,
PZ = peripheral zone.

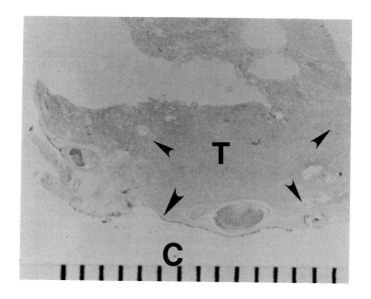

FIGURE 6 (C):   STAGE UB1, non-palpable cancer, Gleason
                grade 2+2 capsular invasion level 2.
                Axial whole mount section shows tumor T
                (arrowheads). Lower arrowhead shows level 2
                capsular penetration.

lesions had a normal or mildly suspicious DRE. Overall,
41% (20/49) of the patients with cancer had a normal or
mildly suspicious DRE (Fig. 13).

     A preliminary study of fine needle aspiration cytology
and histology (22 and 19 gauge) were compared to 14 gauge
histologic cores (N=21). All 19 gauge tissue cores were
adequate histologic specimens. Eighty-six percent (18/21)
of these biopsies were positive compared to 76% (16/21) for
the 14 gauge histology and 67% (14/21) for the 22 gauge
cytology needle. Minimal intraglandular bleeding was noted
under real-time observation. This was in contrast to the
14 gauge histology needle where bleeding was frequently
noted.

     No significant complications were recorded for any of
these patients.

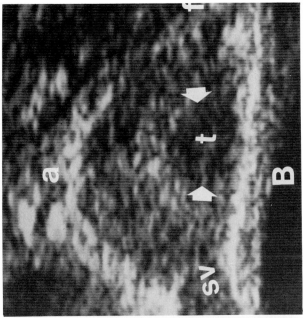
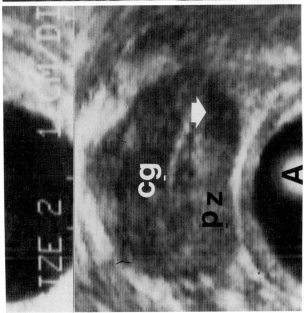

FIGURE 7 (A,B): STAGE UB1, non-palpable cancer, Gleason grade 4+4 capsular penetration level 3.
Axial scan (A) and sagittal scan (B) show tumor t (arrows).

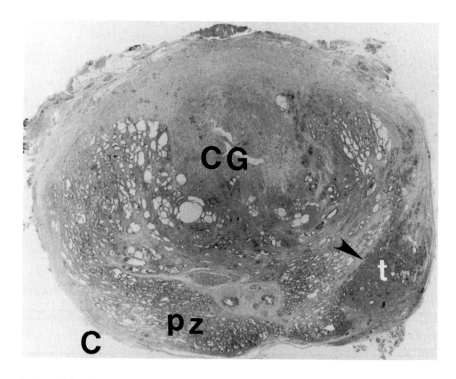

FIGURE 7 (C): STAGE UBl, non-palpable cancer, Gleason
grade 4+4 capsular penetration level 3.
Axial whole mount shows tumor t (arrowhead).

The main groupings of benign biopsies of suspicious
lesions showed that 21% were normal, 29% with glandular
and leiomyomatous hyperplasia, 16% with atypical glandular
or ductal dysplasia, 13% with prostatitis and 21% of others.

PRELIMINARY RESULTS OF AN EARLY DETECTION TRUS VERSUS DRE

Nine patients were found to have prostate cancer, which
is an overall detected prevalence rate of 2.3%, and a
positive predictive value of 29%. When the diagnosis of
atypical glandular hyperplasia, which is considered to be
premalignant, is included, the respective rates are 3.4%
and 42%. The rates for ultrasound alone are 2.1% and 31%

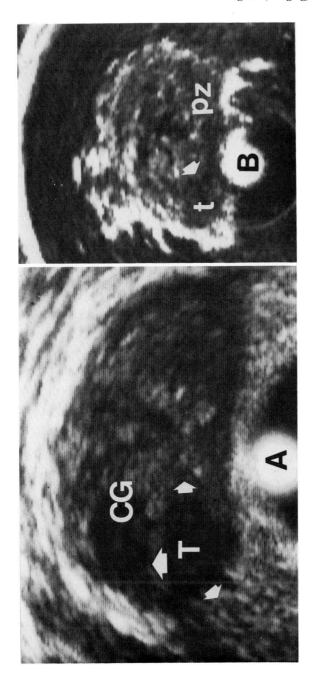

FIGURE 8 (A,B): STAGE UB2, palpable cancer, Gleason grade 2+2 capsular penetration multi-focal lesion, 5mm. Axial scans in vivo (A) and in vitro (B) show tumor (arrows).

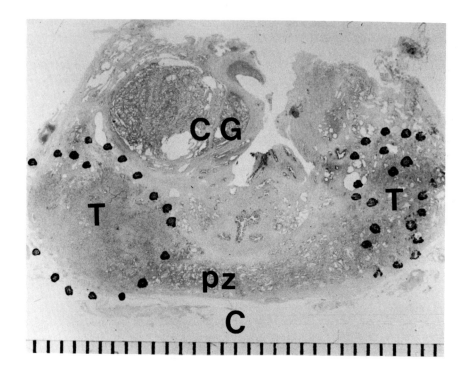

FIGURE 8 (C):   STAGE UB2, palpable cancer, Gleason grade
2+2 capsular penetration multi-focal, 5 mm.
Axial whole mount shows tumor T in the right
peripheral zone (PZ). The tumor T in the
left PZ was not detected by ultrasound. The
adenoma (CG) is hypoechoic on ultrasound (A).

for cancer and 3.1% and 46% for cancer and atypical glandular
hyperplasia. The rates for the digital examination alone
are 1.0% and 27% for cancer, and 1.8% and 47% for cancer and
atypical glandular hyperplasia.

Of a total of 13 lesions detected, there were two
non-curable cancers, seven potentially curable cancers with
average diameters less than 1.5 cm, and four atypical
glandular hyperplasias. Thus 85% (11/13) detected lesions
were potentially curable. Of the potentially curable lesions,
ultrasound detected 100% (11/11), whereas the digital
examination detected 55% (6/11).

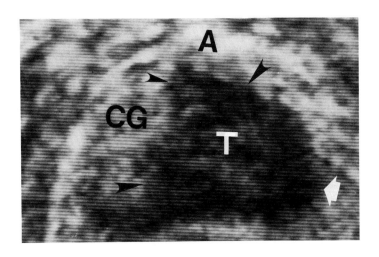

FIGURE 9:   STAGE UB3, non-palpable cancer, Gleason grade 6
            capsular invasion level 2.

     Six of the seven cancers were further evaluated by
surgical intervention and demonstrated excellent correlation
between the ultrasound staging and the final clinical/
histologic staging. The only discrepancy was in the seventh
case. The size of the tumor in the gross specimen was as
predicted by ultrasound, however histologically there was
extra-capsular spread but no evident lymphatic involvement.
This cancer was an undifferentiated adenocarcinoma, Gleason
grade 7. Of the two non-curable lesions, there was proven
nodal involvement in one and bone metastases in the other.
One case, initially called negative by ultrasound, was in
retrospect staged by ultrasound criteria as a UB2 lesion.

     A comparison of DRE with TRUS showed that 46% of
positive biopsies (5 cancers and 1 atypical glandular
hyperplasia) were non-palpable. Conversely, 7.7% of positive
biopsies (1 cancer) were detected by DRE and not by TRUS.
Of the six non-palpable proven lesions, five were considered
potentially curable.

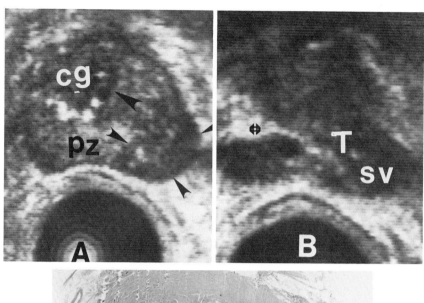

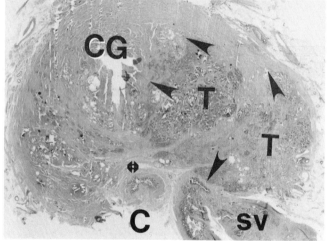

FIGURE 10 (A,B,C):   STAGE UC1 with seminal vesicle extension,
                     palpable cancer, Gleason grade 7 capsular
                     penetration.
                     Axial scans (A,B) show tumor T (arrows)
                     involving the left peripheral zone (PZ)
                     and obliterating the angle between the
                     prostate gland and the seminal vesicle
                     (SV) .⊕ = normal SV angle. Whole section.
                     (C) shows tumor (T) invading left SV
                     (lower arrow).

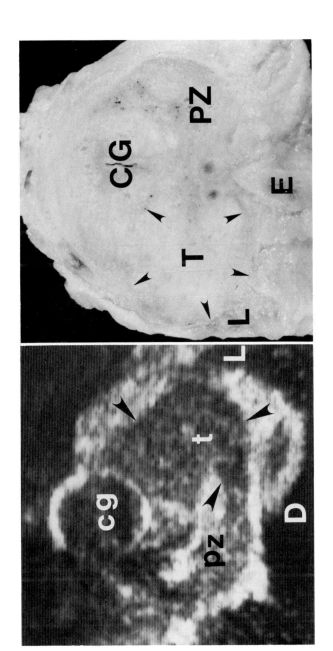

FIGURE 10 (D,E): STAGE UC1 with seminal vesicle extension, palpable cancer, Gleason grade 7 capsular penetration. Axial scan (D) shows tumor (T) extending into central gland (CG). Axial whole mount (E), reversed, shows tumor (T) on the left extending into CG.

FIGURE 11

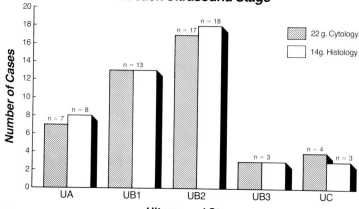

POSITIVE* BIOPSIES
*Comparison of Cytology and Histology
at each Ultrasound Stage*

* Positive = Cancer + Suspicious for Cancer

FIGURE 12

PERCENT POSITIVE* BIOPSIES
*Combined Cytology and Histology
at each Ultrasound Stage*

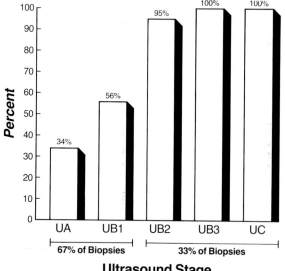

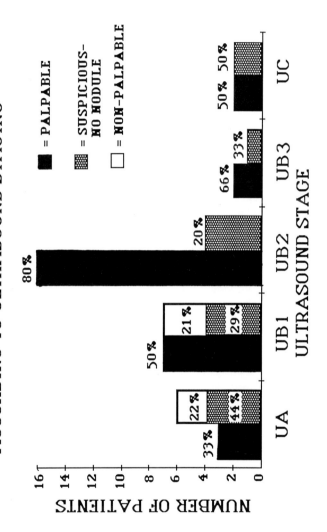

FIGURE 13

DISCUSSION

The previous work of McNeal and others explain many of
the clinical and pathologic observations about cancer of the
prostate (McNeal, 1969; McNeal, 1968; Byar et al, 1972;
Mostofi, Price, 1973).

Our observations show that cancer of the prostate is
anechoic to hypoechoic in appearance and originates in the
peripheral zone. We were unable to detect a difference in
the echogenicity of the smaller anechoic lesions and the
larger more hypoechoic cancers until we imaged at 7.0 MHz.
We believe this anechoic area corresponds with the site of
origin of the cancer. Of all the transducers available to
us, the 7.0 MHz transducer had the best combination of tissue
contrast and resolution. There was no change in echogenicity
of cancer, relative to the degree of tumor differentiation.
Two cancers with a cribiform histologic pattern did have a
slight increase in echogenicity when compared to the other
proven cancers.

Benign hyperplastic tissue has a variable appearance
on ultrasound, ranging from hypoechoic to hyperechoic, and
is located within the central gland. Much of the current
literature suggests that prostate cancer is usually hyperechoic
in appearance and centrally located within the gland (Rifkin
et al, 1983; Fritzsche et al, 1983; Watanabe et al, 1975;
Resnick et al, 1978; Peeling et al, 1979; Rifkin et al, 1986).
We have found that cancers presenting as hyperechoic lesions
within the central gland are mixtures of benign tissue and
infiltrating cancer. In our experience with whole mount
studies and clinical material, this appearance is a late
finding in the continuum of cancer spread. We believe that
the significant overlap in appearance of benign hyperplastic
tissue and benign tissue invaded by cancer accounts for the
low reported specificity of transrectal ultrasound in the
diagnosis of prostate cancer.

Our experience has led to the following ultrasonic-
histologic conclusions regarding tumor growth (Fig. 14):
The smallest tumors 0.0-0.1 cm (UA) are anechoic in appearance
and arise within the tissues of the peripheral zone. These
lesions may involve the inner aspect of the capsule on
ultrasonic imaging. Histologically, all of these lesions
were atypical glandular hyperplasia or well differentiated
adenocarcinoma.

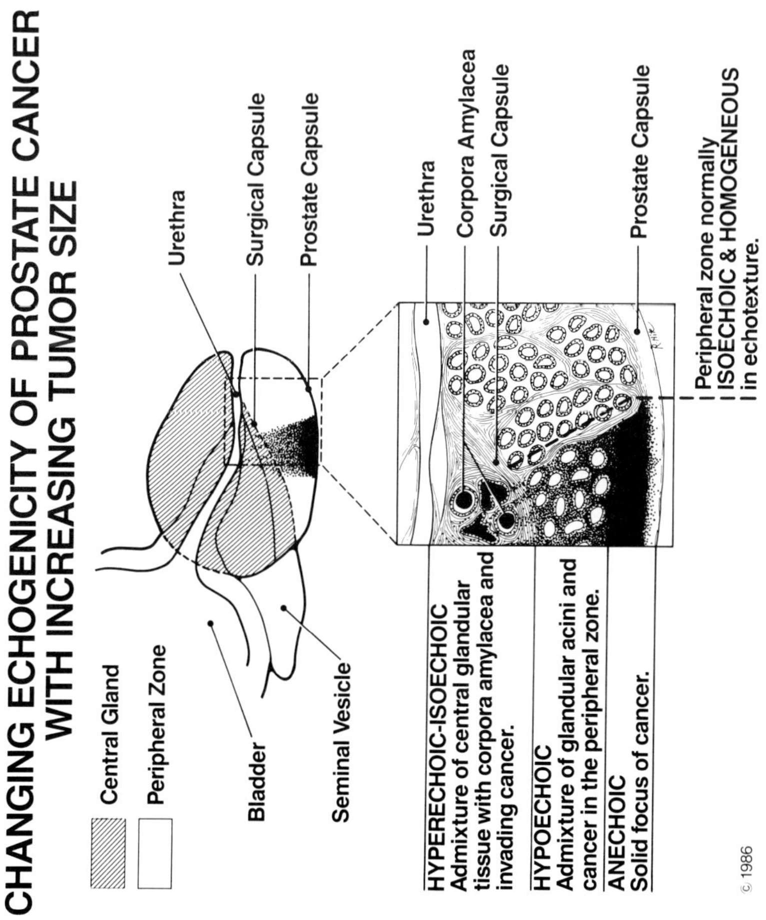

CHANGING ECHOGENICITY OF PROSTATE CANCER
WITH INCREASING TUMOR SIZE

Central Gland

Peripheral Zone

Urethra

Surgical Capsule

Prostate Capsule

Bladder

Seminal Vesicle

Urethra

Corpora Amylacea

Surgical Capsule

Prostate Capsule

Peripheral zone normally
ISOECHOIC & HOMOGENEOUS
in echotexture.

HYPERECHOIC-ISOECHOIC
Admixture of central glandular
tissue with corpora amylacea and
invading cancer.

HYPOECHOIC
Admixture of glandular acini and
cancer in the peripheral zone.

ANECHOIC
Solid focus of cancer.

© 1986

FIGURE 14

As cancers approach 1.5 cm (UB1), they spread in the
subcapsular peripheral zone and retain an anechoic nidus.
The margins however, increase in echogenicity, becoming
hypoechoic in comparison to the normal isoechoic peripheral
zone tissue. Microscopically, this appearance corresponds to
cancer cells surrounding normal glandular elements of the
peripheral zone. Ultrasound demonstrated capsular involvement
in most cases but no extra-prostatic spread was detected.
As the cancer extends centrally, it displaces and subsequently
penetrates the surgical capsule, infiltrating the superficial
aspect of the central gland. Corpora amylacea are found in
glandular acini adjacent to the surgical capsule. These
hyperechoic foci become enveloped by the invading cancer
and account, in part, for the increasing echogenicity of
the advancing cancer margin. Histologically, in both our
clinical series and whole prostate specimens, well
differentiated carcinomas predominated. Four whole mount
specimens, Gleason grade 5, 7, and two of 8 showed microscopic cancer foci outside of the gland.

As the cancers enlarge beyond 1.5 cm (UB2), the
peripheral zone becomes more extensively involved by
hypoechoic neoplasm. The outer aspect of the capsule is
infiltrated and appears thin and irregular. With further
extension into the central gland, the tumor develops a
hypoechoic to hyperechoic appearance, overlapping the
spectrum of the ultrasonic appearance of benign hyperplasia.
Microscopically, there are streaming micro acini of cancer
in the fibromuscular stroma surrounding benign glandular
elements of the hyperplastic tissue. In our clinical series,
there was an increase in the number of less well differentiated
tumors. Our three whole mount cancers over 1.5 cm (UB2) in
diameter demonstrated microscopic extra-capsular spread.
Histologically, these lesions were Gleason grade 4, 5, and
7.

With further glandular involvement (UB3), the contra-
lateral peripheral zone and central gland become involved,
and the ultrasound patterns also change. The anechoic and
hypoechoic foci continue to enlarge, and the tumor involves
the remaining gland, producing a diffuse heterogeneous
pattern. The outer aspect of the capsule appears to be
involved without definite disruption. These cancers were
less well differentiated than the previous stages. The
single whole mount cancer of this stage showed extra-capsular
microscopic spread and a Gleason grade of 7.

The development of an extra-prostatic mass or seminal
vesicle involvement on ultrasound denotes stage UC. The
ultrasound appearance of extra-prostatic extension of cancer
is hypoechoic, apparently a result of the combination of
anechoic cancer and hyperechoic peri-prostatic adipose tissue.
One whole prostate specimen of this stage (UC2) showed a
diffuse heterogeneous hypoechoic pattern with capsular
penetration. Its Gleason grade was 9. A second cancer (UC1)
showed both extra-capsular spread as well as involvement of
the left seminal vesicle. Its Gleason grade was 7.

The importance of detecting small carcinomas cannot be
over-emphasized. The natural history of this disease is
that increasing size accompanies progressive loss of cancer
differentiation and capsular involvement. Concomitantly,
extra-prostatic spread becomes increasingly likely.

Scott and co-workers found that tumor size greater
than 1.0 cm was accompanied by extension of tumor outside of
the capsule in 84% of their cases. They also noted a
progressive loss of differentiation with increasing tumor size
(Scott et al, 1969). McNeal has published similar statistics
with only 6% of tumors 0.1 to 1.0 cc's associated with
involvement of the outer aspect of the capsule, whereas 80%
of tumors 1.0 to 1.5 cc's have outer capsular segments
involved (McNeal, 1969). Culp and Meyer found a significant
decrease in survival time with tumors 1.5-2.0 cm in diameter
(Culp, Meyer, 1973).

The findings of our present ultrasound study are in
agreement with radical prostatectomy studies. In our
whole mount series, four cancers 1.0-1.5 cm in average
diameter (UB1) with Gleason grades greater than 5, showed
extra-capsular spread. The potential for curability
appears to be dependent on at least three crucial factors -
size of lesion, degree of tumor differentiation and capsular
integrity. Though our series is small, a Gleason grade over
5 may have prognostic significance. All cancers greater
than 1.5 cm in diameter, in our whole mount specimens,
demonstrated microscopic spread outside of the capsule.
Larger cancers were more likely to involve or perforate the
outer portions of the capsule.

The biopsy yield for cytology and histology were
approximately equal. These studies should not be thought
of as separate for both are complementary. The cytologic

needle has a dual function which it performs well. This is evident from our results where 4/5 (80%) cases with negative histology and positive cytology were subsequently proven to be cancer. In 11 cases with cytologic insufficient tissue, the six corresponding histology were cancer. The cytologic needle can successfully target lesions for guiding of larger bore needles and to sample the lesion itself.

Grouping of our lesions according to ultrasound staging allowed us to correlate our results with those suggested by the DRE. DRE's considered normal or mildly suspicious occurred predominately in the lesions less than 1.5 cm in diameter. Over half of this group (57%) of potentially curable lesions would have either been overlooked or followed for restudy and not immediately biopsied. The classic urologic description for prostate cancer should be revised in view of our current ultrasound findings. Recent articles in the urologic literature stress that even marginal DRE findings warrant cytologic needling of the prostate for cancer (Chodak, 1986). TRUS has the ability to properly evaluate the equivocal DRE and when positive findings are suggested, to guide thin needles to the area for biopsy. In our screening program, 46% of the positive biopsies were in fact non-palpable of which 5/6 (83%) were potentially curable. The results from our screening program and needle study confirm the fact that lesions less than 1.5 cm in diameter are not well evaluated by the DRE.

In hope of detecting potentially curable prostate cancers, we must combine the equivocal DRE's with TRUS. By doing this, we may be able to effect a lowering of the death rate (25,000/year) for this ubiquitous cancer.

CONCLUSIONS

Cancer of the prostate originates within the tissue of the peripheral zone and is anechoic to hypoechoic in echo-texture. Small lesions are predominately well differentiated.

Transrectal ultrasound can detect cancer of the prostate before it reaches 1.0 to 1.5 cm in average diameter. We found microscopic extra-prostatic spread as well as progression of the neoplasm to less degrees of histologic differentiation with tumors greater than 1.5 cm in average diameter.

The potential for curability appears to be dependent on at least three crucial factors - size of lesion, degree of histologic differentiation and capsular integrity.

Ultrasound guidance of thin needle biopsies is the diagnostic method of choice for the definitive evaluation of early prostate cancer.

There was close agreement of the ultrasound size of the tumor and the size at gross sectioning. Because of this, it is possible to predict extent of local glandular involvement with ultrasound, allowing for accurate staging.

Because of the ability of transrectal ultrasound to demonstrate small, non-palpable, potentially curable cancers, it has promise for being utilized as a screening modality.

REFERENCES

Bryan PJ, Butler HE, Lipuma JP, Haaga JR, El Yousef SJ, Resnick MI, Cohen AM, Malviva VK, Nelson AD, Clampitt M, Alfidi RJ, Cohen J, Morrison SC (1983). NMR scanning of the pelvis: Initial experience with a 0.3 T system. AJR 141:1111-1118.

Byar DP, Mostofi FK and the Veterans Administration Cooperative Urological Research Group (1972). Carcinoma of the prostate: Prognostic evaluation of certain pathologic features in 208 radical prostatectomies. Cancer 30:5-13.

Ca: A cancer journal for clinicians (1985). Cancer Statistics, pp 19-35. Published by the American Cancer Society in New York.

Chodak GW, Walk V, Parmes E, Watanabe H, Ohe H, Saitoh M (1986). Comparison of digital examination and transrectal ultrasonography for the diagnosis of prostate cancer. J Urol 135:951-954.

Culp OS, Meyer JJ (1973). Radical prostatectomy in the treatment of prostatic cancer. Cancer 32:1113-1118.

Dahnert WF, Hamper UM, Eggleston JC, Walsh PC, Sanders RC (1986). Prostatic evaluation by transrectal sonography with histopathologic correlation: The echopenic appearance of early carcinoma. Radiology 158:97-102.

Emory TH, Reinki DB, Hill AL, Lange PH (1983). Use of CT to reduce understaging in prostatic cancer: Comparison with conventional staging techniques. AJR 141:351-354.

Franks LM (1954). Latent carcinoma of the prostate. J Path Bact 68:603-616.

Fritzsche PJ, Axford PD, Ching VC, Rosenquiest RW, Moore R (1983). Correlation of transrectal sonographic findings in patients with suspected and unsuspected prostatic disease. J Urol 130:272-274.

Golimbu M, Morales P, Al-Askari S, Shulman Y (1981). CAT scanning in staging of prostatic cancer. Urology 18: 305-308.

Helpap B (1980). The biological significance of atypical hyperplasia of the prostate. Virchows Arch [Path Anat] 387 (3):307-317.

Kastendieck H, Altenahr E, Husselmann H, Bressel M (1976). Carcinoma and dysplastic lesions of the prostate. Z Krebsforsch 88:35-54.

Lee F, Gray JM, McLeary RD, Lee F Jr, McHugh TA, Solomon MH, Kumasaka GH, Straub WH, Borlaza GS, Murphy GP (1986). Prostatic evaluation by transrectal sonography: Criteria for diagnosis and early carcinoma. Radiology 158:91-95.

Lee F, Gray JM, McLeary RD, Meadows TR, Kumasaka GH, Borlaza GS, Straub WH, Lee F Jr, Solomon MH, McHugh TA, Wolf RM (1985). Transrectal ultrasound in the diagnosis of prostate cancer: Location, echogenicity, histopathology and staging. Prostate 7:117-129.

Lee F, Littrup PJ, McLeary RD, Kumasaka GH, Borlaza GS, McHugh TA, Soiderer MH, Roi LD (1986). Needle aspiration and core biopsy of prostate cancer: Comparative evaluation using biplane transrectal ultrasound guidance. Accepted for publication by Radiology.

Ling D, Lee JKT, Heiken JP, Balfe DM, Glazer HS, McClennan BL (1986). Prostatic carcinoma and benign prostatic hyperplasia: Inability of MR imaging to distinguish between the two diseases. Radiology 158:103-107.

McNeal JE (1969). Origin and development of carcinoma in the prostate. Cancer 23:24-34.

McNeal JE (1983). The prostate gland: Morphology and pathobiology. 1983 Monographs in Urology 4:3-33.

McNeal JE (1968). Regional morphology and pathology of the prostate. AM J Clin Path 49:347-357.

Mostofi FK, Price EB (1973). "Tumors of the male genital system." Washington DC, Armed Forces Institute of Pathology, pp 196-252.

Peeling WB, Griffiths GJ, Evans KT, Roberts EE (1979). Diagnosis and staging of prostatic cancer by transrectal ultrasonography. A preliminary study. Br J Urol 51:565-569.

Resnick MI, Willard JW, Boyce WH (1978). Ultrasonic evaluation of prostatic nodule. J Urol 120:86-89.

Rickards D, Gowland M, Brooman P, Mamtora H, Blacklock NJ, Isherwood I (1983). Computed tomography and transrectal ultrasound in the diagnosis of prostatic disease - A comparative study. Br J Urol 55:726-732.

Rifkin MD, Friedland GW, Shortliffe L (1986). Prostatic evaluation by transrectal endosonography: Detection of carcinoma. Radiology 158:85-90.

Rifkin MD, Kurtz AB, Choi HU, Goldberg AB (1983). Endoscopic ultrasound evaluation of the prostate using a transrectal probe: Prospective evaluation and acoustic characterization. Radiology 149:265-271.

Schmidt JD (1985). Confirming the diagnosis, evaluating the extent of disease. "Cancer of the Prostate - A Desk Reference," Dominus Publishing Co., Inc. pp 17-24.

Scott R Jr, Mutchnick DL, Laskowski TZ, Schmalhorst WR (1969). Carcinoma of the prostate in elderly men: Incidence, growth characteristics and clinical significance. J Urol 101:602-607.

Sheldon CA, Williams RD, Fraley EE (1980). Incidental carcinoma of the prostate: A review of the literature and critical reappraisal of classification. J Urol 124:626-631.

Stamey TA (1983). Cancer of the prostate: An analysis of some important contributions and dilemmas. 1983 Monographs in Urology 4:68-92.

Watanabe H, Igari D, Tanahashi Y, Harada K, Saitoh M (1975). Transrectal ultrasonotomography of the prostate. J Urol 114:734-739.

Whitmore WF Jr (1956). Symposium on hormones and cancer therapy: Hormone therapy in prostate cancer. AM J Med 21:697-713.

The Use of Transrectal Ultrasound in the Diagnosis and
Management of Prostate Cancer, pages 111–123
© 1987 Alan R. Liss, Inc.

TECHNIQUES IN THE FINE NEEDLE ASPIRATION BIOPSY OF THE PROSTATE

Paul Ray

Division of Urology, Cook County Hospital and
the Univeristy of Illinois College of Medicine,
Chicago, Illinois 60612

ABSTRACT   In general,   aspiration cytology of
the prostate has not been a frequently used
technique, in part because all too often
there has been a poor yield of cells for
cytologic evaluation.   The objective of this
investigation was to evaluate various needle
designs and techniques for obtaining specimens and making slides.   Cadaver prostates
and surgical specimens were used to evaluate
a series of 22 gauge aspiration needles.
Cytology slides were fixed and stained with
either Papanicolaou or hematoxylin and eosin
stain.   Coded slides were assigned a score
representing the number of fields (magnification X 40) covered.   The angle of the
bevel or the size of the side-port (0.030
inch long and 0.01 inch deep or 0.045 inch
long and 0.01 inch deep) did not significantly affect the results.   However, the presence
of the side-eye on a control spinal needle or
an existing Franzen aspiration needle significantly improved the yield of cells (P
<.05).   Frosted and non-frosted slides were
evaluated as well as other techniques for
making smears.   In conclusion, an outline for
making cytologic slides for aspirations of
the prostate is presented.

Present address: Chairman, Division of Urology
Cook County Hospital, Chicago, Illinois 60612

INTRODUCTION

Encouraging data that the potential exists for the earlier detection of prostatic cancer is accompanied, not unexpectedly, with some controversy (Lee et al., 1985). For the first time, the questions of the relative value of detection of cancer of the prostate in very early stages of its development are being raised. Ultrasound of the prostate seems likely to play an important role. Fine needle aspiration (FNA) with ultrasound as well as without ultrasound is attractive because of its ease and decreased morbidity. Yet, aspiration cytology of the prostate is not widely accepted in the United States. There are two basic reasons for this. The first is that the yield of cells was too poor for pathologists to read. Too often the cytology report returned with the comment that the specimen was insufficient. The second reason may be due to the relative inexperience of pathologists reading prostatic aspiration.

We postulated that if the design of the needle used for aspiration cytology of the prostate could be changed to increase the yield of cells, the technique would be less "technician dependent" and this method would gain wider acceptance. There are reports that needle design can alter the yield of aspirated tissue (Andriole et al., 1983). Numerous reports indicate aspiration cytology of the prostate to be as accurate as core biopsy (Chodak et al., 1984, Hosking et al., 1983, Ljung et al., 1986) with less morbidity (Kaufman et al., 1982, Esposti 1966). This report will detail the data regarding the development of the Ray and Lee-Ray needle as well as other parameters to obtain good aspiration specimens.

MATERIALS AND METHODS

Phase I.

Prostates obtained from cadaver and surgical specimens were used to evaluate a series of 22

gauge aspiration needles (Table 1).
Twenty-two gauge spinal needles and the currently marketed Franzen needles were compared to Franzen needles with a side port and a thin walled 22 gauge needle with long and short bevels (LB,SB) and side-ports (SP) either .030 or .045 inches long.

TABLE 1.
NEEDLE DESIGN INVESTIGATED

---

22 GAUGE SPINAL NEEDLE

FRANZEN
FRANZEN WITH SMALL SIDE-PORT

SPINAL NEEDLE, LONG BEVEL, SIDE-PORT .045 INCH(LB)
SPINAL NEEDLE, LONG BEVEL, SIDE-PORT .030 INCH(LB)
SPINAL NEEDLE, SHORT BEVEL, SIDE-PORT .045 INCH(SB)
SPINAL NEEDLE, SHORT BEVEL, SIDE-PORT .030 INCH(SB)

The slides were made by aspirating from one lobe of the prostate. The order of each needle was random and the same technique was used for each needle. The order of needle was then reversed and the procedure repeated from the other lobe. The slides were fixed immediately in 95% ethanol and stained with Papanicolaou or hematoxylin and eosin stains.

Coded slides were assigned a score representing the number of fields (magnification X 40) covered. An analysis of variance was used to determine a probable difference. Differences between individual groups were determined by the T statistic.

Phase II.

The second phase of the evaluation compared the highest scoring needle, a 22 gauge thin walled needle, 3 1/2 inches long with a clear plastic hub and a rectangular side-port opposite the bevel 0.030 inches long a 0.010 inch deep, to a 3 1/2 inch long spinal needle. A spinal needle was selected because previous to the development of the side-ported needle, the spinal needle and the Franzen needle were both currently used for aspiration cytology, and the score was significantly higher for the spinal needle.

RESULTS

Phase I.

The mean score of the 3 major groups of needle designs are illustrated in Table 2.

TABLE 2.
COMPARISON OF NEEDLE DESIGN IN CADAVER
AND SURGERY PROSTATE SPECIMEN

NEEDLE	MEAN SCORE ± SD	P VALUE TO SPINAL NEEDLE	P VALUE TO FRANZEN
22 GAUGE SPINAL NEEDLE	2.09 + .41		
FRANZEN	1.21 + .40	<.01*	
FRANZEN WITH .030 INCH SP	2.21 + .54		<.01
LB SP .045 INCH	2.78 + .85	<.05	<.001
LB SP .030 INCH	2.71 + .68	<.05	<.001
SB SP .045 INCH	2.75 + .58	<.05	<.001
SB SP .030 INCH	2.75 + .72	<.05	<.001

F = 13.42
* = probabilty value <.01 lower score to spinal needle

It is interesting to note that the widely

used Franzen needle had the lowest score. The 22 gauge spinal needle, another needle commonly used for aspiration cytology of the prostate, was significantly better than the Franzen with a P value of <.005 when compared to the spinal needle. The length of the bevel did not have any significant effect on the yield of prostatic cells, nor did the size of the side-port. Interestingly, the modification of the existing Franzen by the addition of a side-port significantly (p <.003) improved the yield of cells.

Phase II.

The results of the test needles on cadaver and surgical prostate specimens lead to the development of a 22 gauge, thin walled needle, 3 1/2 inches long with a clear plastic hub and a retangular side-port 0.030 inches long and 0.010 inches deep. A comparison was made to the next best type of needle currently used by urologists for fine needle aspiration of the prostate, a 22 gauge spinal needle. A newly designed formable finger guide, illustrated in Figure 1, was used to accurately place transrectally the needle to the desired point of aspiration. The same technique was used in aspiration. The results (Table 3) show the experimental needle significantly improved the yield of cells as compared to the next best available needle.

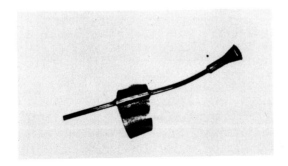

FIGURE 1. The transrectal formable finger guide for use with the 3 1/2 inch 22 gauge thin walled aspiration needle.

TABLE 3.
COMPARISON OF NEEDLES

NEEDLE	MEAN SCORE	P VALUE
22 GAUGE SPINAL NEEDLE	1.30 ± 0.16*	
EXPERIMENTAL	2.20 ± 0.29	< 0.05

*Standard Error Of The Mean

DISCUSSION

Needle.

The wide clinical acceptance of aspiration cytology requires that the pathologists/ cytologists have an adequate and interpretable specimen. The experiments outlined above lead to the development of a 3 1/2 inch long (9 cm) aspiration needle and formable finger guide. A similar needle 20 cm long, the Lee-Ray aspiration needle for aspiration with ultrasound guidance is now available.*

Fixative.

An adequate but poorly preserved cytological specimen does not aid the number of successful interpretations. There are numerous "tricks" to optimizing a cystology slide. In performing an aspiration, one must initially decide if the cytological specimen is to be air-dried or fixed. If fixed, is it to be fixed in 95% ethanol or by spray fixative? The preference of the pathologist should be considered regarding these choices. If any type of fixative is used, the slide should be

*Cook Urological, Spencer, Indiana

fixed within seconds after the smear, to prevent drying. If the slides are dipped into ethanol, they should stay in that solution 15 to 20 minutes, after which they can be removed and allowed to dry. The ethanol solution should not be used for another patient's slide because some cells shed from a previous slide may be cancerous, and become adherent to a patient's slide who has only a benign prostate, causing a wrong diagnosis. The ethanol between patients should be discarded or filtered with No. 2 filter paper. If the convenience of spray fixative is desired, there are a number of products available, all of which seem to work for some individuals, at a wide range in price. Again, it is important to fix the slide immediately after the smear with the spray and to spray evenly to avoid washing the cells to the edges of the slide. With the kind of fixative that we use, the spray is held 3-4 inches from the slide. The Pathologist should be aware of the fixative used since a few fixatives require re-hydration before staining.

Slides.

There are two basic types of slides available, clear sides which are frosted at one end or completely frosted slides. The latter are more expensive, but helpful if one has difficulty in the technique of "smearing"; i.e., with the edge of one slide, spreading the one drop of aspiration evenly over the slide to cover approximately 2/3 of the surface. If there seems to be a consistent problem with excessive fluid at the end of the slide, the increased surface area of the frosted slide easily solves the problem. However, there is an artifact caused by the rough surface of this slide, particularly observed in the sheets of cells seen in benign prostatic hyperplasia. The difference in appearences is illustrated in Figure 2 and 3. The sheets may have a shreaded appearance with the frosted slides.

Movement.

The art of aspiration has been practiced many ways. Some practitioners have avocated a rapid

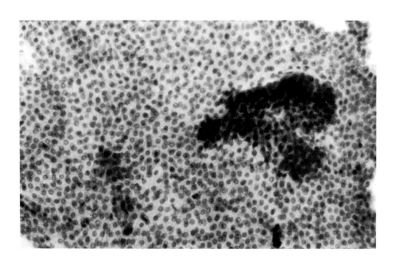

FIGURE 2.   BPH seen in sheets of cells

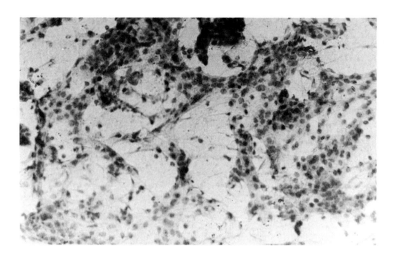

FIGURE 3.   BPH with shreading artifact seen with a frosted slide.

back and forth movement, perhaps .5 to 1.5 cm in distance 10 times or several times that, others have recommended continuing this cell-gathering motion 20 or 30 seconds. Our philosophy is that we wish only to aspirate the specific suspicious areas so far as possible, and reduce "contamination" as much as feasible from blood (which also clots in the needle) or other prostatic cells which may dilute the important cells on the slide. Therefore, the tip of the needle is placed into the suspicious area and suction is applied to the 5 cc mark in the syringe. The typical back and forth motion is made .5 to 1 cm until the specimen is seen collecting in the clear plastic hub. More specimen is not necessary if properly gathered. By choice, we will repeat this procedure 3 times. More than this adds to the discomfort of some patients and increased dilution of the specimen by blood.

Pressures.

Figure 4 illustrates the decrease of pressure (ΔP) in mmHg generated as plunger is pulled back. In addition to the volume of air displaced, the negative pressure is dependant on the initial volume of the system as expressed in the relationship:

$$\frac{(S)(X)}{V_o} = \frac{1}{\dfrac{760}{\Delta P} - 1}$$

where ΔP is negative pressure, $(S)(X)$ is the volume displaced as the plunger is pulled back and V_o is equal to the initial volume of the system. The normal aspirating system with the Ray or Lee-Ray needle have an initial volume of .09 and .10 ml respectively. As ΔP approaches 760 mmHg asymptocially , there is little is to be gained by pulling the plunger back further than 5 cc.

General Technique of Aspiration.

Before beginning the aspiration, the slides and fixative should be placed on a nearby table. Care should be made that the correct surface of

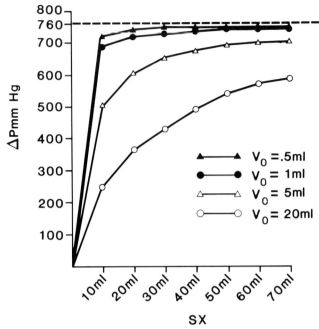

FIGURE 4. The change in negative pressure
(Δ P) in relationship to changing volume of the
system (S)(X). The effect of the initial volume
V_o is seen in four conditions:

the slide is facing up. The patient is placed in
position (usually lithotomy) for the procedure
(Figure 5 and 6). The needle is placed on the
syringe with the plunger pushed in to ensure
minimal initial volume. Either by ultrasound
guidance or transrectally, the tip of the needle
is placed in the center of the lesion. Suction is
applied and in the manner described previously
until specimen is seen in the clear plastic hub;
however avoid if possible diluting the aspiration
with blood.
    Some specimen is lost when the plunger is
gently allowed to return to its initial position
to equalize the pressure. If the aspiration
appears especially fluid, loss of the specimen can
be minimized by disingaging the needle from the
syringe or pulling the plunger out to 6 cc, where
a small hole has been bored in the barrel of the
syringe, thereby equalizing the pressure.

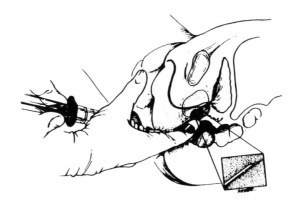

FIGURE 5. Transrectal finger guided
aspiration (FNA).

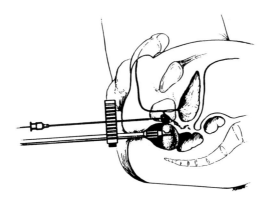

FIGURE 6. Transperineal aspiration with
ultrasound guidance.

The needle is removed from the tissue and
with the side-port against the slide, a drop is
placed on the slide. If there is more specimen
left in the needle, the second drop is placed on a
second slide. This is done to avoid covering the
entire slide with the smear. If the slide is not
to be air- dried, the slide must be immediately
fixed. If the aspiration was bloody, then the

needle should be washed in 5-10 ml saline and sent
for cell block since there is a possibility that
cells will become trapped in a blood clot that
often forms in the needle under in such conditions.

CONCLUSION

The addition of a side-port in the needle
significantly improved the yield of cells when
compared to similar needles without a side-port.
The 22 gauge, thin walled Ray or Lee-Ray needle is
a first step in improving the yield of cells.
Attention to the methodologies in making and
fixing the slide should greatly improve the number
of interpretable slides and be of benefit to our
patients.

ACKNOWLEDGMENTS

I wish to thank Dr. Vera Ray for her expert
reading of the cytology slides, Dr. Patrick Guinan
for his insights and Dr. Marc Boukerche for help-
ing me in interpreting Boyle's Law.

REFERENCES

Andriole JG, Haaga JR, Adams RB and Nunez C
    (1983). Biopsy needle characteristics assessed
    in the laboratory. Radiology 148:659-662.
Chodak GW, Bibbo m, Straus FH, Wied GL (1984).
    Transrectal aspiration biopsy versus transper-
    ineal core biopsy for the diagnosis of carcinoma
    of the prostate. J of Urol 132:480-482.
Esposti PL (1966). Cytologic diagnosis of
    prostatic tumors with the aid of transrectal
    aspiration biopsy. A critical review of 1,100
    cases and a report of morphologic and
    cytochemical studies. Acta cytol 10:182-186.

Hosking DH, Paraskevas M, Hellsten OR, Ramsey EW (1983). The cytological diagnosis of prostatic cancinoma by transrectal fine needle aspiration. J of Urol 129:998-1000.

Kaufman JJ, Ljung BM, Walther P, Waisman J (1982). Aspiration biopsy of prostate. Urology 19:587-591.

Lee F, Gray JM, McLeary RD, Meadows TR, Kumasaka GS, Borlaza GS, Straub WH, Lee F Jr., Solomon MH, McHugh TA and Wolf RM (1985). Transrectal ultrasound in the diagnosis of prostate cancer: location, echogenicity, histopathology, and staging. The Prostate 7:117-129.

Ljung BM, Cherrie R, Kaufman JJ (1986). Fine needle aspiration biopsy of the prostate gland: a study of 103 cases with histological followup. 135:955-958.

The Use of Transrectal Ultrasound in the Diagnosis and
Management of Prostate Cancer, pages 125–131
© 1987 Alan R. Liss, Inc.

HISTOLOGIC AND CYTOLOGIC DIAGNOSIS OF PROSTATIC CARCINOMA BY
ULTRASOUND-GUIDED NEEDLE BIOPSY

Manfred H. Soiderer, M.D.

Department of Pathology, St. Joseph Mercy
Hospital, P.O. Box 995, Ann Arbor, Michigan   48106

HISTORY

The idea of sampling an organ by needle is said to have
been first applied at Memorial Hospital for Cancer in New
York City in 1930. Martin and Ellis developed the method to
avoid open tissue biopsy on the one hand and assessment of
the extent of neoplasm by clinical examination alone on the
other hand (Martin and Ellis, 1930). Large bore needles
(gauge 16) were used; the material was smeared and stained
by hematoxylin and eosin. Tissue cores were fixed in formalin and processed in the usual manner. Russell Ferguson,
a urologist at the same institution, applied the technique
to the prostate gland using an 18 gauge needle and the
transperineal approach (Ferguson, 1930 and 1937). The core
needle biopsy technique continued to be developed to its
present state of the art but aspiration cytology entered a
long slumber in this country. In Europe, primarily in
Sweden, aspiration biopsy of multiple organs was further
developed using small-bore needles which yielded material to
be smeared, stained, and examined cytologically rather than
by tissue section. Instruments for fine needle aspiration
of the prostate gland were described by 1960 by Franzen,
Giertz, and Zajicek (Franzen et al, 1960). Fine needle
aspiration biopsy has taken hold now in this country. In
our Department of Pathology, we currently interpret aspirated material from lung, liver, pancreas, kidney, lymph
nodes, salivary glands, breast, thyroid gland, skin, soft
tissue (including retroperitoneum), mediastinum, and prostate gland.

METHODS FOR LOCALIZING PROSTATIC LESIONS

The most common method has been digital examination in spite of its inability to detect small lesions and the accessibility of only a portion of the gland. Ultrasound is capable of detecting lesions as small as 3-5 mm and also provides direct guidance for the biopsy needle (Lee, 1986). In order to determine the success rate, 100 needle biopsies performed under ultrasound guidance were analyzed. This was the first group of 100 lesions in which a core needle biopsy and a fine needle aspiration (for cytology) were carried out on the same patient and in which adequate material was obtained by at least one biopsy technique.

Results of 100 Consecutive
Ultrasound Guided Biopsies

	Core Biopsies	Aspirations	Total
Carcinomas	45	39	47
Suspicious	0	4 *	0

* The four lesions suspicious by fine needle aspiration were carcinomas proven by core biopsy.

Four carcinomas were found only by core biopsy and two carcinomas were present only in fine needle aspirates. The total number of carcinomas in 100 ultrasound guided aspirates was 47.

In order to increase the sensitivity of the fine needle aspirations, cell blocks are prepared in the following manner:

1. After the smears for cytology have been made, the needle or needles are rinsed in physiologic saline.
2. The saline suspension is centrifuged and the supernatant is discarded.
3. Three or four drops of outdated blood bank plasma are added to the cell button (which is usually invisible) and the cells are resuspended.
4. Two or three drops of topical thrombin (5000 units of tropical thrombin from the pharmacy diluted with sterile distilled water to a concentration of 500 units per cc) are added to the mixture with slight agitation. A clot forms readily.
5. The clot is removed from the tube by inversion or a wooden stick, stained with eosin for ease of

identification, wrapped in lens paper, and placed in formalin for fixation as tissue.

6. The clot is processed as surgical tissue, embedded in paraffin, sectioned in the usual manner (usually at two levels), and stained with hematoxylin and eosin.

RESULTS OF THE CELL BLOCK TECHNIQUE

Thirty-five fine needle aspirates which revealed carcinoma had a concomitant cell block. Of these 35 cell blocks, 21 contained neoplasm. In fact in three of the 21 cell blocks, only the cell block material revealed carcinoma. In other words, without the cell blocks, three of the 35 aspirates would have been falsely negative.

HISTOLOGIC CRITERIA FOR THE DIAGNOSIS OF ADENOCARCINOMA

The best defined and probably the most reliable criteria are those developed by Gleason (Gleason, 1977) . The 5 Gleason patterns describe the range of histologic appearances from well differentiated to moderately differentiated and to poorly differentiated but in a precise manner. Briefly the patterns are:

1. Well defined tumor margins. Single separate round glands of medium size, closely packed. Minimal stromal invasion.
2. Less definite tumor margins. Single separate rounded glands with more variability and of medium size. Glands separated by stroma up to one gland diameter.
3. Poorly defined tumor margins. Single separate, more irregular glands or rounded masses of cribriform or papillary epithelium. Gland size is small, medium or large. Glands spaced more than one gland diameter apart, rarely packed. Moderate stromal invasion.
4. Ragged infiltrating tumor margins. Fused glandular masses. Glands small, dark or hypernephroid.
5. Poorly defined tumor margins. Few or no glands; very small if present. Rounded masses and cords of tumor cells infiltrating the stroma.

The Gleason tumor grade is a combination of the dominant pattern and the secondary pattern. The application of the Gleason system to core biopsies is not entirely satisfactory particularly if the amount of neoplasm is scanty and if the Gleason score is low (Garnett et al, 1984), (Babaian and Grunnow, 1985), (Mills and Fowler, 1986). However it may be useful to use Gleason patterns (not scores) as descriptive terms in addition to identifying the neoplasm as well, moderately or poorly differentiated.

There are other grading systems the most recently published being the M.D. Anderson tumor grading system.

CYTOLOGIC CRITERIA FOR THE DIAGNOSIS OF ADENOCARCINOMA VS. BENIGN LESIONS

1. Cytologic features of benignancy

> Well demarcated borders around large cell sheets
> Uniform cells in an orderly arrangement
> Uniform, usually round nuclei
> Relatively low cellularity
> Inflammatory cells may or may not be present
> Epithelial cells from normal prostate gland are
>   identical to those from a hyperplastic gland

2. Criteria for inflammatory lesions

> Acute prostatitis: Neutrophils
>   Small number of lymphocytes
>   and histiocytes
>   Debris
>   Often high cellularity

> Chronic prostatitis: Histiocytes
>   Lymphocytes
>   Plasma cells
>   Scattered epithelial cells
>   Small cell clusters rather
>   than large sheets
>   Cytoplasmic borders more
>   indistinct
>   Some nuclear variability

3. Criteria for adenocarcinoma

The Gleason system does not lend itself to the interpretation of fine needle aspirates as smears, although attempts are made periodically. It is is possible to distinguish well differentiated carcinoma from poorly differentiated carcinoma, but mixed patterns make it more complex.

> Well differentiated adenocarcinomas:

>> Microglandular structures
>> More non-cohesive cell clusters
>> Indistinct cell boundaries

Variation in nuclear size
Macronucleoli

Moderately differentiated adenocarcinoma:

Scattered single malignant cells
Small non-cohesive tumor fragments
Greatly reduced cytoplasm with ill-defined
  cytoplasmic borders
Marked nuclear variability
Macronucleoli

Poorly differentiated adenocarcinoma:

Naked nuclei, sometimes bizarre
Small, non-cohesive clusters
Indistinct cytoplasmic borders
Usually little cytoplasm
Increased nuclear/cytoplasmic ratio
Macronucleoli

4. Pitfalls in the cytologic diagnosis of prostatic
    carcinoma

Seminal vesicle cells and ejaculatory duct epithelium may exhibit malignant features and must be
recognized for what they are; they generally contain
yellow cytoplasmic granules or clumps. Rectal epi-
thelial cells usually present no problem. In extremely well differentiated adenocarcinomas, the nucleoli
may not be as prominent and the neoplastic sheets may
be more benign appearing.

The qualities of the aspirate and of the prepared
cytologic smears are crucial. There must be immediate
fixation to avoid air-drying artifact. The aspirated
material must be properly spread in a non-traumatic
way. It is essential that there be communication and
cooperation between the radiologist, urologist and
pathologist.

USES OF FINE NEEDLE ASPIRATION AFTER THE INITIAL DIAGNOSIS
OF PROSTATIC CARCINOMA

1. Reassessment of the prostate gland after radiation
    treatment

After successful therapy the prostatic aspirate is
usually sparse. There may be metaplastic squamous
cells, histiocytes, and scattered inflammatory cells.
The core biopsy will often have an atrophic appearance

although there will be stromal fibrosis and atypical
reactive changes in endothelial cells.

2.   Retroperitoneal lymph node aspiration biopsy

The cytologic criteria for smears and the histologic criteria for cell blocks are the same in retroperitoneal lymph node aspirates as they are in prostatic aspirates. One pitfall must be carefully avoided. The lymphangiography contrast material in retroperitoneal lymph nodes evokes a granulomatous reaction
consisting of single and multinucleated histiocytic
giant cells with a distinct nucleolus in most nuclei.
These cells may resemble adenocarcinoma. If sufficient
material is available, the problem can be resolved by
the application of the immunoperoxidase stain for prostatic specific antigen.

SUMMARY, CONCLUSIONS, AND RECOMMENDATIONS

In a group of 100 consecutive patients with an abnormal
ultrasound picture of the prostate gland, forty-seven were
found to have adenocarcinoma by core and/or aspiration biopsy. Others report yields of 25% (Chodak et al, 1986), 29%
(Chodak and Schoenberg, 1984), and 30% (Kline, 1985) by conventional assessment of the prostate gland and without the
use of ultrasound, for an average yield of 28% in these
three series. The almost double yield in our patient population most likely is attributable to the ability of ultrasound to identify carcinoma and to localize it for biopsy.
The accuracy of core biopsies and fine needle aspirates is
approximately equal; in combination they provide the most
accurate results.

REFERENCES

Babaian RJ, Grunnow WA (1985). Reliability of Gleason
grading system in comparing prostate biopsies with total
prostatectomy specimens. Urology 25:564-7.
Chodak GW, Steinberg GD, Bibbo M, Wied G, Straus FS II,
Vogelzang NJ, Schoenberg HW (1986). The role of transrectal aspiration biopsy in the diagnosis of prostatic
cancer. J Urol 135:366-7.
Chodak GW, Schoenberg HW (1984). Early detection of prostate cancer by routine screening. JAMA 252:3261-4.
Ferguson RS (1937). Diagnosis and treatment of early
carcinoma of the prostate. J Urol 37:774-782.
Ferguson RS (1930). Prostate Neoplasms: their diagnosis by

needle puncture and aspiration. Am J Surg 9:507-511.

Franzen S, Giertz G, Zajicek J (1960). Cytological diagnosis of prostatic tumors by transrectal aspiration biopsy: A preliminary report. Br J Urol 32:193.

Garnett JE, Oyasu R, Grayhack JT (1984). The accuracy of diagnostic biopsy specimens in predicting tumor grades by Gleason's classification of radical prostatectomy specimens. J Urol 131(4):690-3.

Gleason DF (1977). Histologic grading and clinical staging of prostatic carcinoma. In Tannenbaum M (ed): Urologic Pathology: The Prostate, p. 171. Philadelphia, Lea and Febiger.

Kline TS (1985). Guides to Clinical Aspiration Biopsy: Prostate. New York-Tokyo, Igaku-Shoin.

Martin HE and Ellis EB. Biopsy by needle puncture and aspiration. Ann Surg 92:169,1930.

Mills SE and Fowler JE Jr. Gleason histologic grading of prostatic carcinoma. Correlations between biopsy and prostatectomy specimens. Cancer 57(2):346-9, 1986.

Lee F (1986). Personal Communication.

The Use of Transrectal Ultrasound in the Diagnosis and
Management of Prostate Cancer, pages 133–142
© 1987 Alan R. Liss, Inc.

PREVENTIVE ONCOLOGY PROJECT FOR PROSTATIC CANCER

Hiroki Watanabe

Department of Urology, Kyoto Prefectural
University of Medicine
Kawaramachi-Hirokoji, Kyoto, Japan 602

PREVENTIVE ONCOLOGY

Medicine can be divided into two categories,
namely, therapeutic medicine and preventive medicine, with the large majority of current medicine
is devoted to therapeutic medicine. However,
therapeutic medicine for cancer now faces big
barriers involving incredible effort still to be
made. In this situation, the importance of preventive oncology is generally being recognized
more and more.

Preventive oncology consists of two areas,
namely, primary and secondary prevention. The
former is the prevention of the generation of disease, which is achieved by avoiding risk factors
revealed through epidemiologic investigations.
The latter is the prevention of the progression of
disease, which is achieved by detecting patients
in the pre-clinical stage and treating them before
onset.

GROWTH MODEL OF PROSTATIC CANCER

At the beginning of the preventive oncology
project for prostatic cancer, we made a hypothesis
on the growth model of prostatic cancer (Fig. 1).
According to the multiple hit theory of cancer, it
was considered that risk factors for prostatic

cancer work in two steps. When the first factor
acts on the normal prostate, latent cancer may be
generated. When the second factor is added to
this, clinically manifest cancer may be formed.

As well known, latent cancer is a phenomenon
specially seen in prostatic cancer. This consists
of small cancer foci a few mm in diameter with no
expansion, invasion or metastasis and is thought
to be basically different from clinically manifest
cancer. According to autopsy studies, this phenomenon be detected in approximately 20% of the
general male population in the higher age range in
any countries. Although no treatment is necessary
for this condition, much evidence indicates that a
limited number of latent cancers will be activated
at some moment and will change into clinically
manifest cancers.

The question is how shall we intervene in
this growth process of prostatic cancer in our
preventive oncology project? It may be not ad-
visable to intervene at the latent cancer stage,
because the subjects to be dealt with will be too
many, resulting in too much cost and social disruption.

For that reason, we decided that our project
should intervene at two points; one at the point
between latent cancer and the pre-onset of clinical cancer as primary prevention, and another at
the point between the pre-onset and the onset of
clinical cancer as secondary prevention. The former may be achieved through awareness of how to
reduce or cancel the risk factors for cancer and
the latter through mass screening for the early
detection of cancer.

PRIMARY PREVENTION

For primary prevention, we made an epidemiological study to clarify the high risk group for
prostatic cancer[1]. An original questionnaire,
consisting of 111 questions, was designed in 1976.
A case-control study by matched-pair analysis was

conducted from 1976 to 1981 on 100 prostatic cancer cases and 100 controls matched for age within
1 year and for residence in the same prefecture.
The cases and controls were interviewed by well
trained urologists. Statistically significant results from the study will be summarized in Table 1.

For occupation and income, risk factors were:
No involvement with an administrative job, contact
with dyes at work, lack of military service and
present annual income less than 1,200,000 yen.
These bracket factors present an image of blue-
collar people in the lower income.

For diet, risk factors were: Not taking sea
food everyday, not taking green and yellow vege-
tables everyday, preference for spices and preference for salty things. This may indicate a
Western diet rather than a traditional Japanese
one.

As for sexual habits, risk factors were:
Marriage younger than at age 24, marriage lasting
for more than 40 years, first sexual intercourse
at less than age 19, frequency of sexual intercourse more than once per month from age 15 to 20,
frequency less than once per month from age 61 to
70, and an early cessation of sexuality. These
can be summarized as an active sexuality in younger years and an inactive sexuality in advanced
years. This pattern of sexual history may become
more distinct with the display for relative risk
on the frequency of sexual intercourse in 10 year
steps (Fig. 2).

We have published information regarding the
risk factors of prostatic cancer for people's
awareness in newspapers, magazines, on television
and in films as widely as possible. According to
our estimate, awareness has been achieved for a
total of over 10 million people in Japan up to
1984.

SECONDARY PREVENTION

Systematic activity for mass screening for prostatic cancer as the secondary prevention has not really begun yet even in Western countries, mainly because no suitable diagnostic means for the purpose of screening has been available.

We originally developed transrectal sonography (TRS) in 1967 and found that this new diagnostic means is suitable for the screening of prostatic cancer and benign prostatic hypertrophy. For that reason, we organized a new mass screening program for prostatic diseases, using transrectal sonography as the primary study of the program in 1975[2].

TRS is a simple and non-invasive examination with an excellent diagnostic ability, indicating a sensitivity of 96.6% and a specificity of 81.8% for prostatic cancer[3]. It takes less than 3 minutes to carry out for each person including preparation time.

The system of the mass screening program is as follows: As a rule examinees are limited to males over 55 years of age. Each examinee is first asked to supply details of his medical history by a questionnaire and then examined using TRS for the primary study. In some necessary occasions digital palpation is combined. Sonograms are evaluated carefully, taking the data from the questionnaire into consideration. When the findings warrant it, some screened subjects are requested to submit to a secondary study which consists of an ordinary urological examination including digital palpation, measurement of residual urine, X-ray procedures, and/or prostatic needle biopsy, if necessary.

Model trials of the screening system were initially performed on 180 males between January, 1975[2], and April, 1977[4]. In the next stage, we advanced to field trials on 145 males from November, 1977, to September, 1979, in two small towns near Kyoto[5]. In all of these trials the equipment necessary for the studies was transported by motor vehicle and set up at each location.

Based on the data obtained in these trials, a proto-type mobile unit for the primary study was developed in January, 1980[6]. This was followed by the development of a practical mobile unit, the "Dolphin", in December, 1980[7]. The name "Dolphin" was chosen because of the connection with that animal's use of ultrasound for communication.

The floor area of the bus is about 8 m^2, with an operation console in the center where two chair-type transrectal scanners are fixed one on either side. During the examination of one person on one side, the next person is in preparation on the other side. There is no undressing area inside the unit because examinees only have to lower their trousers to the knee for examination. The capacity of the unit is approximately 20 examinees per hour, which comes to some 150 examinees every day.

Up to March, 1986, 5,070 males from various areas in Japan were submitted to the mass screening program. The final diagnoses are given in Table 2. After the primary study, the prostates of 1,484 males were diagnosed ultrasonically as abnormal. By the secondary study, 1,179 males (23.3%) were diagnosed as having benign prostatic hypertrophy and 24 males (0.5%) as having prostatic cancer. The detection rate of 0.5% is significantly high as compared with other screening systems e.g. for gastric cancer (0.1%), uterine cancer (0.15%) or breast cancer (0.06%)[8].

In 46% of the patients in whom prostatic cancer was detected, the malignancy belonged to Stage B. This rate for detection in the early stages is much larger than that in general urological clinics, indicating a proportion between 10 and 20%.

Some typical cases will be demonstrated. The sonogram shown on Fig. 3 is of a case having a tiny nodule of cancer in the left lobe of the prostate.

The section is slightly asymmetric and a hypoechoic area is seen in the left lobe.

Fig. 4 is also a case of prostatic cancer in
Stage B. A deformity of the section is observed.

Following our project, a mass screening for
prostatic cancer has been started recently in
several areas in Japan and is obtaining similar
results. The system is thus being appreciated
very much even in Japan, where the incidence of
the disease is only one tenth of that in Western
countries. There is no doubt that this type of
intervention would be very effective especially in
Western countries. We strongly recommend such
countries to consider the possibility of adopting
the system.

REFERENCES

1) Mishina T, Watanabe H, Araki H, Nakao M (1985).
   Epidemiological study of prostatic cancer by
   matched-pair analysis. Prostate 6: 423-436.
2) Watanabe H, Saitoh M, Mishina T, Igari D,
   Tanahashi Y, Harada K, Hisamichi S (1977).
   Mass screening program for prostatic diseases
   with transrectal ultrasonotomography. J Urol
   117: 746-748.
3) Watanabe H, Date S, Ohe H, Saitoh M, Tanaka S
   (1980). A survey of 3,000 examinations by
   transrectal ultrasonotomography. Prostate 1:
   271-278.
4) Watanabe H, Saitoh M, Ohe H, Tanaka S, Itakura
   Y (1977). A mass screening program for prostatic diseases by means of transrectal ultrasonotomography in two homes for the aged.
   Proc Jap Soc Ultrasonics Med 32: 123-124.
5) Watanabe H, Saitoh M, Ohe H, Tanaka S, Itakura
   Y, Yamanaka Y, Ohta Y (1978). A first ex-
   periment of field mass screening program for
   prostatic diseases by means of transrectal
   ultrasonotomography. Proc Jap Soc Ultrasonics
   Med 33: 151-152.
6) Watanabe H, Ohe H, Mishina T, Tanaka S, Kaneko
   Y, Ohta Y (1980). A mass screening program

for prostatic diseases (1st report)---Develop-
ment of a prototype mobile unit for mass
screening of prostatic diseases---. Proc Jap
Soc Ultrasonics Med 36: 381-382.

7) Watanabe H, Ohe H, Inaba T, Itakura Y, Saitoh
M, Nakao M (1984). A mobile mass screening
unit for prostatic disease. Prostate 5:
559-565.
8) Watanabe H (1985). Secondary prevention in
preventive oncology. Oncologia 12: 54-68.

TABLE 1. High risk group of prostatic cancer

Occupation and income

	Odds ratio
No involvement with administrative job*	3.24
Contact with dyes at work	11.00
Lack of military service*	2.23
Present annual income less than ¥1,200,000	1.70

Diet

Not taking sea food everyday*	1.97
Not taking green and yellow vegetables everyday	1.97
Preference for spices*	1.78
Preference for salty things*	1.94

Sexual habit

Marriage younger than age 24*	2.50
Marriage lasting for more than 40 years	1.57
First sexual intercourse at less than age 19	3.37
Frequency of sex. int. over 1/month from age 15 to 20*	2.19
Frequency of sex. int. less than 1/month from age 61 to 70*	2.17
Earlier cessation of sexuality*	3.57

*p < 0.05   others : p < 0.1

TABLE 2. Result of mass screening
(January, 1975 — March, 1986)

Examinee	5070
Average age	65.2 y.o.
Cases for secondary study	1484 (29.3%)
Final diagnosis	
BPH Stage I	930 (18.3%)
BPH Stage II	249 (4.9%)
Prostatic cancer	24 (0.5%)
Prostatitis	63 (1.2%)
Miscellaneous	77 (1.5%)

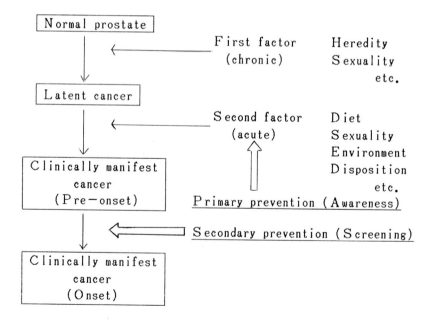

Fig. 1. Growth model of prostatic cancer (Watanabe)

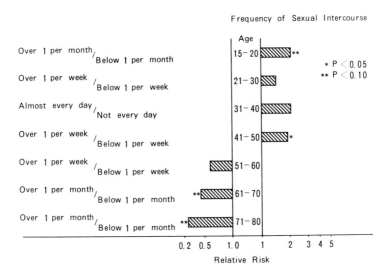

Fig. 2.   Frequency of sexual intercourse and
          relative risk for prostatic cancer.

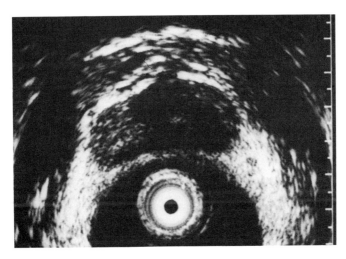

Fig. 3.   Prostatic cancer in Stage B₁.
          Hypoechoic area in the left lobe.

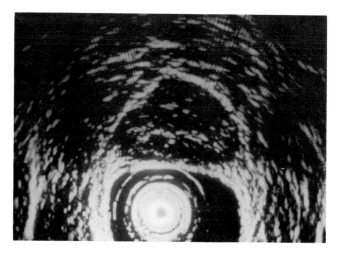

Fig. 4.   Prostatic cancer in Stage B_2.
          Deformity of the prostatic section.

The Use of Transrectal Ultrasound in the Diagnosis and
Management of Prostate Cancer, pages 143–152
© 1987 Alan R. Liss, Inc.

TRANSPERINEAL I-125 SEED IMPLANTATION IN PROSTATE CANCER
GUIDED BY TRANSRECTAL ULTRASOUND

Soren Torp-Pedersen, M.D., H. H. Holm, M.D.,
Peter J. Littrup, M.D.

Departments of Ultrasound (S.T.P., H.H.H.), Herlev
Hospital, 2730 Herlev, Denmark; Department of
Radiology (P.J.L.), St. Joseph Mercy Hospital,
P.O. Box 995 Ann Arbor, Michigan 48106.

Potentially curative therapy of localized cancer of
the prostate can be obtained with either radical prostatectomy, external beam or interstitial radiation therapy.
The final choice of therapy is dependent upon the patient's
age, physical condition and acceptance of associated side
effects, as well as the therapeutic traditions of each
institution.

With interstitial therapy, a high radiation dose can
be delivered to the prostate with minimal damage to
surrounding tissues. Iodine-125 is considered to be an
ideal isotope for implantation due to its half-life of 60
days and a half-value layer of only 1.7 cm in human tissue
(Catalona, 1984). These characteristics permit a relatively
slow growing cancer to receive sustained irradiation, yet
limiting the dose to the adjacent rectal wall. Following a
staging lymphadenectomy to rule-out D1 disease, conventional
seed implantation is performed by inserting needles into
the prostate under digital guidance (Whitmore et al, 1972).
The seeds should be evenly distributed throughout the gland
to account for the multifocal nature of adenocarcinoma of
the prostate. Additional seeds are often placed in and
around the palpable nodule to assure an adequate tumoricidal
dose.

Transperineal seed implantation utilizing transrectal
ultrasound (TRUS) guidance was developed in 1982 at Herlev
Hospital, Copenhagen (Holm et al, 1983). This technique
allows for improved accuracy of seed placement and spares
the patient a major surgical procedure. In the following,

appropriate staging procedures, a planning session, and
seed implantation will be described. Due to copyright
constraints, the results of individual patient follow-up
from the Herlev Hospital series will not be included.

STAGING

In the initial series at Herlev, the TNM staging system
was used and To-2, No, Mo cancers were selected for
interstitial therapy. Preoperative evaluation for distant
metastases included a bone scan, acid phosphatase and
ultrasound examination of the liver. TRUS evaluation of
the prostate was used to confirm the absence of capsular
penetration and local extension. Ipsilateral extra-peritoneal
pelvioscopy (Hald, Rasmussen, 1980) was then performed to
assess local nodal involvement and further lymphadenectomy
was avoided.

The ultrasound staging system for prostate cancer
proposed by Lee, et al, represents a superior evaluation of
intraglandular tumor volume and potential histologic extent
of tumor (Lee et al, Accepted for Publication in Radiology).
The accurate biopsy and follow-up of suspicious lesions may
lead to the identification of earlier, smaller cancers.
Pathologic studies have demonstrated limited capsular
penetration with tumors less than 3.0 cc in volume (McNeal
et al, 1986), which correlates with approximately 1.44 cm
in average diameter by TRUS measurements. By limiting
interstitial therapy to tumors less than 1.5 cm in average
diameter (stages UA and UB1), the efficacy of this modality
may be improved.

PLANNING PROCEDURE

The patient is placed in the lithotomy position and the
Bruel & Kjaer 7 MHz axial probe is introduced into the rectum.
The probe is held in place by a special fixture which has
been mounted onto the operating table (Fig. 1). This fixture
allows for precise movement control of the probe along the
x, y and z axes.

The actual needle matrix is electronically simulated
as a dot matrix overlay on the monitor (Fig. 2). The
fixture is then adjusted so that the bottom row of the dot

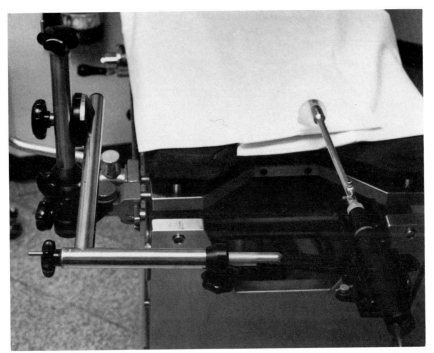

FIGURE 1:   Implantation   fixture mounted on operating table
with the axial probe in place.

matrix closely approximates the posterior border of the
prostate from base to apex. Starting at the base, sectional
images of the prostate are obtained at 5 mm intervals
throughout the gland. At each step, the prostate is outlined
with a light pen and the volume is obtained by the summation
of each slice area.

The activity and distribution of the I-125 seeds are
calculated to match the shape and volume of the gland. A
cylindrical model is developed using only those dots within
the outlined borders of the gland in the sequential ultrasound
images (Fig. 3). The implantation needles are then individually loaded with I-125 seeds and Teflon spacers according
to their predetermined distribution within the cylindrical
model. Each needle is labeled to match its position on
the implantation matrix and the appropriate scan plane for

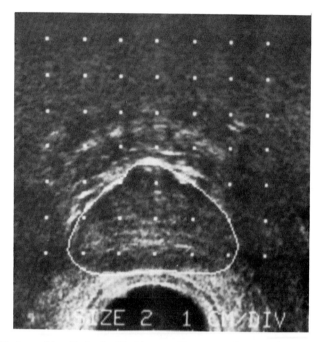

FIGURE 2:   Simulated (dot) needle matrix projected onto
the axial scan with the prostate outlined for
voluming. The bottom row of dots is adjusted
to approximate the posterior border of the
prostate.

insertion.

IMPLANTATION PROCEDURE

    The percutaneous implantation is performed in general
or spinal anesthesia. The patient is placed in the same
lithotomy position used in the planning procedure to avoid
altering the shape of the prostate from variable contraction
of the pelvic muscles.

    The axial probe is placed in the rectum of the patient
and mounted in the fixture. With the electronic dot matrix
on the monitor, the fixture is manipulated until the bottom

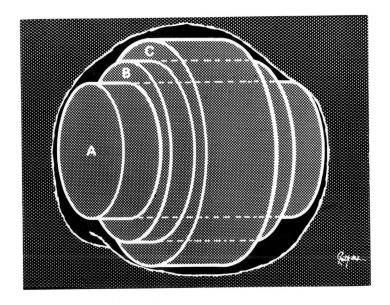

FIGURE 3:   Cylindrical implantation model defining three
            scan plans for needle insertion. The inner
            cylinder (A) begins at the cranial-most scan
            plane.

row of dots approximates the posterior border of the prostate
as in the planning procedure.

    The scrotum is lifted anteriorly and the perinuem prepped
and draped in the usual fashion. The sterile needle matrix
is then mounted on the rectal tube of the probe (Fig. 4).
The axial probe is positioned at the cranial-most scanning
plane at the base of the prostate. The matrix is positioned
approximately 3 cm from the perineum. An empty needle is
inserted into the prostate through the matrix in order to
stabilize the gland.

    The appropriately labeled needles for this scanning
plane are then inserted into the prostate through their
corresponding holes on the matrix. The correct position
of each needle is verified on the monitor +/- 2 mm from its
corresponding dot). Incorrect needle position can be

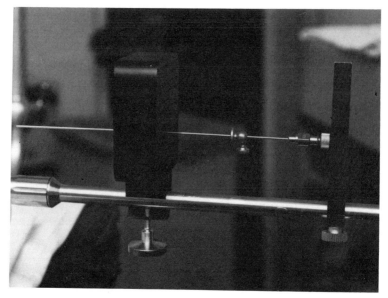

FIGURE 4:   Implantation matrix mounted on axial probe with needle and stopper in place.

adjusted by altering the position of the needle bevel on re-insertion and/or appropriate retraction of the skin to further guide the needle.

One by one, the needles are emptied by swinging a stopper behind the stylet of each needle and retracting the needle over the stylet. A row of seeds and spacers are thus extruded by the stylet into the prostate (Fig. 5). Each needle is checked with a geiger counter to assure that no seeds remain in the needle. The scanner is then retracted to the next scanning plane for insertion and the procedure is repeated.

The number of seeds and corresponding punctures depend upon the volume and shape of each prostate. The total procedure usually takes an hour: 30 minutes to adjust the fixture and 30 minutes for the actual implantation. No obvious hematoma or increase in total glandular volume has been noted after implantation.

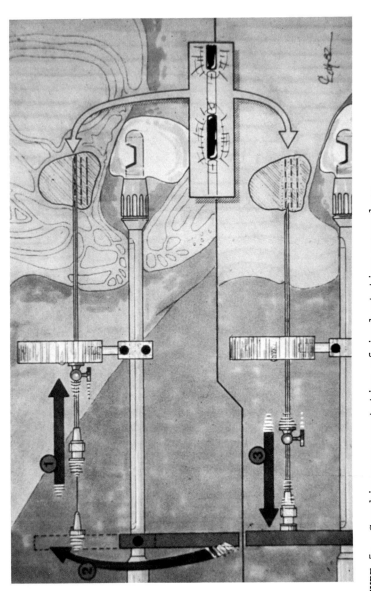

FIGURE 5: Graphic representation of implantation procedure. Step 1: A loaded needle is inserted into the prostate. Step 2: The stopper is swung up behind the needle stylet. Step 3: The needle is withdrawn over the stylet, depositing the I-125 seeds and Teflon spacers.

During the first post-operative day, the patient voids through a filter in order to catch any seeds expelled through the urethra. The average hospital stay has only been two days for the actual implantation procedure.

Biplane radiographs (Fig. 6) and/or pelvic CT show the resultant distribution of the seeds from which corresponding isodose curves can be constructed. If any "cold" spots in the prostate are then found, the implantation procedure may be repeated with insertion of additional seeds in the desired areas. The prostate receives a total of approximately 160 Gy of interstitial irradiation. In the Herlev series, this was supplemented with 40 Gy of external beam irradiation to cover any occult metastases to the iliac lymph chain.

FOLLOW-UP

Patients at Herlev received TRUS evaluation and voluming of the prostate at three and six month intervals during the first two years. A decrease in gland volume was seen in nearly all cases. Biopsy of the initial tumor region was performed each year to assess for viable residual tumor.

We believe that TRUS guided transperineal implantation assures more accurate needle placement than the standard "open" technique and is relatively atraumatic. Furthermore, the improved symmetry of seed placement and close proximity to the capsule ensure a high uniform dose to all prostatic tissue.

With early detection programs and improved tumor voluming techniques, smaller cancers may be selected for therapy. After a sufficient trial period has demonstrated no obvious tumor involvement on pelvic lymphadenectomy (or pelvioscopy), these operative procedures could be obviated for small tumors, ie. less than 3.0 cc in volume. Localized prostate cancer may thus be diagnosed, staged and definitively treated utilizing TRUS and transperineal interstitial therapy.

REFERENCES

Catalona WJ (1984). "Prostate Cancer". Orlando: Grune and Stratton, Inc., pp 130.

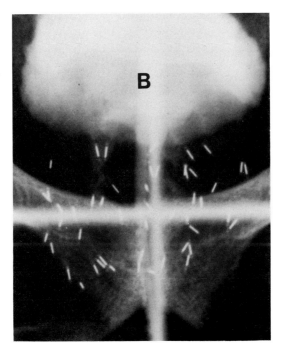

FIGURE 6:   Antero-posterior radiograph of the pelvis showing
            symmetrical seed distribution. The bladder (B)
            has been filled with contrast.

Hald T, Rasmussen F (1980). Extra peritoneal pelvioscopy:
  A new aid in staging of lower urinary tract tumor. A
  preliminary report. J Urol 125:245-248.
Holm HH, Juul N, Pedersen JF, Hansen H, Stroyer I (1983).
  Transperineal 125-iodine seed implantation in prostatic
  cancer guided by transrectal ultrasonography. J Urol 130:
  283-286.
Lee F, Littrup PJ, McLeary RD, Kumasaka GH, Borlaza GS,
  McHugh TA, Soiderer MH, Roi LD (1986). Needle aspiration
  and core biopsy of prostate cancer: Comparative evaluation
  using biplane transrectal ultrasound guidance. Accepted
  for publication in Radiology.
McNeal JE, Kindrachuk RA, Freiha FS, Bostwick DG, Redwine EA,
  Stamey TA (1986). Patterns of progression in prostate
  cancer. The Lancet 11:60-63.

Whitmore WF Jr, Hilans B, Grabstald H (1972). Retropubic implantation of iodine 125 in the treatment of prostatic cancer. J Urol 108:918-920.

The Use of Transrectal Ultrasound in the Diagnosis and
Management of Prostate Cancer, pages 153–159
© 1987 Alan R. Liss, Inc.

THE U.S.A. EXPERIENCE: DIAGNOSIS AND FOLLOW-UP OF PROSTATE
MALIGNANCY BY TRANSRECTAL ULTRASOUND

Robert P. Huben

Department of Urologic Oncology, Roswell Park
Memorial Institute
Buffalo, New York, 14263

INTRODUCTION

Although the prostate gland is readily accessible to
digital examination, this method of determining the nature
and extent of disorders affecting the prostate is notoriously inaccurate. Diagnostic imaging of the prostate with
currently available techniques is similarly problematic.
Transrectal ultrasonography is emerging as a major diagnostic tool in determining the presence and nature of diseases
of the prostate gland. The application of transrectal ultrasound in routine follow-up of patients with prostate
cancer may provide a more objective means of determining
response to therapy. The question of the correlation between local and systemic response to treatment in advanced
prostate cancer is largely unanswered. The purpose of the
present discussion is to review the reported results of
transrectal ultrasonography in the diagnosis and follow-up
of prostate cancer in the United States.

DIAGNOSTIC APPLICATIONS

The future role of transrectal ultrasound in the
treatment of prostate cancer depends on its ability to
first diagnose the disease. The normal prostate gland appears as a triangular or semilunar structure with multiple
fine homogenous echoes which are believed to represent the
acoustic interfaces created by the periurethral glands
(Spirnak and Resnick, 1984). Prostate cancer is characterized by asymmetric enlargement of the gland and alteration of

the pattern of the internal echoes. The nature of the
changes in the relative density of the internal echoes within the prostate gland which characterize prostate cancer
is a matter of conflict and controversy. Early studies
reported that prostate cancer caused an increase in internal
echoes (Spirnak and Resnick, 1984). However, later reports
suggest a relative hypoechogenicity or an indeterminate
pattern in prostate cancer (Lee et al., 1985; Burks et al.,
1986; Dähnert et al., 1986). Lee and Gray were among the
first to suggest the hypoechogenicity which may be the more
typical appearance of prostate cancer (Lee and Gray, 1985).
Lee and associates have presented convincing ultrasonographic and pathologic correlation of hypoechoic areas within
the prostate and the presence of prostate malignancy (Lee
et al., 1985). A predominately echopenic pattern in prostate cancer was also reported by Dähnert and associates
(Dähnert et al., 1986). Histopathologic correlation in a
group of 49 patients who underwent radical prostatectomy
revealed that prostatic carcinoma presented as an echopenic lesion in 54% of specimens, as slightly hypoechoic
area in 22%, and isoechoic in 24% of cases. A later study
by these authors showed that all echogenic foci within
prostates containing tumors represented prostatic calcifications (Dähnert et al., 1986). A somewhat more confusing
report is that of Burks and associates (Burks et al., 1986).
The authors reported considerable overlap in the sonographic
characteristics of benign and malignant lesions. Mixed
echogenicity, consisting of any combination of hyper-,
hypo-, and iso-echogenicity, was the most common pattern
in cancer (65%), but represented only 28% of the benign
conditions. Hyperechogenicity was present in 55% of benign
lesions and 58% of malignant lesions when considering the
components of mixed lesions. Hypoechogenicity was found to
be much less frequent in benign disease (24%) than in malignant disease (58%). A comparison of digital examination
and transrectal ultrasonography in the diagnosis of prostate cancer has recently been reported (Chodak et al.,
1986). In a group of 22 patients with known prostate cancer, tumor was suspected correctly in all of 5 patients
with clinical Stage C disease, while false negative results
occurred in 3 of 17 patients with Stage B disease. Two of
the 3 false negatives were seen in patients with tumors less
than 1 cm in diameter. The overall sensitivity of transrectal ultrasonography was 86%, but the specificity was only
41%. The authors also suggested the limited role of transrectal ultrasonography as a screening procedure in the

United States because of its low positive predictive value.

MONITORING TREATMENT RESPONSE

A method of determining the objective response to
therapy of prostate cancer, whether hormonal, chemothera-
peutic, or radiotherapeutic, has remained a major area of
controversy in the treatment of prostate cancer. Bone
scans are, by necessity, the most commonly used method of
monitoring response to therapy in metastatic disease.
Problems in the interpretation of serial bone scans, particularly early in the course of treatment, have been well
documented. Transrectal ultrasonography may represent a
practical and reproducible means of determining treatment
response. Parameters of response include the nature and
timing of changes in prostate configuration following treatment. Changes in the morphology of the prostate following
treatment are decrease in prostatic size and resumption of
a more normal shape, reformation and thickening of the capsule, diminution of the extent of extracapsular extension,
and normalization of the seminal vesicles (Fujino and
Scardino, 1985). Varying treatment modes result in charac-
teristic intervals between initiation of treatment and maximal normalization of the prostate as determined by transrectal ultrasonography. Maximal reduction in the size of
the prostate usually occurs by 9 months after radiotherapy
and by 3 months following chemotherapy (Fujino and Scardino,
1985). Following hormonal therapy, decrease in prostatic
size occurs within 6 months and subsequent changes are then
minimal (Spirnak and Resnick, 1984). The changes seen after
initiation of estrogen therapy are similar to those after
orchiectomy, but are slower to occur (Resnick et al., 1980).

In our experience, transrectal ultrasonography has been
a useful method of determining local recurrence following
either radical prostatectomy or radical cystectomy. Palpation alone has very limited value following these procedures because of the induration and scarring which normally occur. This technique also facilitates subsequent
needle biopsy or aspiration for cytology to confirm the
diagnosis by providing ultrasound guidance. Similarly, we
have used transrectal ultrasound to monitor response to
therapy for other tumors originating in the prostate, including a leiomyosarcoma, a lymphoma, and a bulky transitional cell carcinoma of the prostate. Interestingly, the

predominant echo pattern in these other tumors of the
prostate was also hypoechoic.

Parameters of response to treatment are poorly defined. As mentioned, normalization of the size and configuration of the prostate are generally seen in those patients responding favorably to treatment. It has been suggested that the two most sensitive measures for monitoring
the primary tumor are the calculated volume of the prostate
and the integrity of the prostate capsule (Fujino and
Scardino, 1986). The rate and degree of tumor reduction
following definitive radiation therapy correlated significantly with the histologic grade of the tumor, and poorly
differentiated tumors decreased most rapidly. There was
also a correlation with the outcome of treatment, while
tumor stage did not correlate with the degree of tumor reduction. In their series of 19 patients, there was a
significant reduction in the mean size of the prostate at
6 months post radiation (20%), with a maximum decrease of
about 35% at 9 to 15 months.

OTHER DIAGNOSTIC AND THERAPEUTIC APPLICATIONS

Another diagnostic application of transrectal ultrasonography involves its use as a method of directing aspiration or biopsy of small but suspicious prostatic lesions
as shown by ultrasound. In fact, the problem of sampling
error has been a real problem in developing ultrasonographic and pathologic correlation. What is seen on the screen
may not be what comes out in the biopsy. A number of methods of coupling the ultrasound image with directed biopsy
have already been described, and that is an area which is
likely to engender further research and more advanced, reproducible, and accurate results.

Perhaps the most promising application of transrectal
ultrasonography is in the clinical staging of patients with
biopsy-proven carcinoma of the prostate. Current staging
methods are notoriously inaccurate in determining pathologic stage, and most surgical series have shown a high rate
of understaging of localized prostate cancer. Cystoscopy
and digital examination are the usual means of assessing
tumor stage, while computerized tomography and other
radiographic techniques have limited value in staging
prostate cancer. Transrectal ultrasonography prior to

radical prostatectomy affords a splendid opportunity to develop ultrasonographic and pathologic correlation.

Several studies have shown that transrectal ultrasonography is a useful adjunct in staging localized prostate cancer (Resnick et al., 1980; Pontes et al., 1985). Problems in interpretation involve the presence or absence of capsular involvement and the ultrasonographic appearance of seminal vesicle involvement. It may be unrealistic to expect that a diagnostic study would demonstrate a microscopic phenomenon, but further correlative studies may show more obvious ultrasonographic changes or patterns which are highly suggestive of capsular or seminal vesicle involvement. However, transrectal ultrasonography already provides a useful and practical means of distinguishing surgically amenable lesions from those which are not.

Therapeutic applications of transrectal ultrasonography at present evolve around its use in directing implantation of radioactive seeds into the prostate. Problems with uneven or haphazard seed implantation has been cited as a cause of failure in implantation techniques used in the treatment of prostate cancer. As in the area of guided biopsy or aspiration techniques, further developments in the therapeutic application of transrectal ultrasonography may be imminent.

SUMMARY

Our own experience, and a review of the American literature, suggests a number of areas in the diagnosis and follow-up of prostate cancer in which transrectal ultrasonography is a useful adjunct. Accurate clinical staging in patients with known prostate cancer is an obvious area in which this technique had ready and practical impact. Its performance prior to radical prostatectomy should facilitate further ultrasonographic and histopathologic correlation. This imaging modality may be coupled with other devices to guide in a precise manner subsequent biopsy or implantation. Further collaborative efforts in this area are likely to result in a number of new and ingenious methods of mapping the prostate gland for further diagnostic or therapeutic intervention with pinpoint accuracy.

At present, one of the most useful applications of transrectal ultrasound is in determining local response to

therapy, whether hormonal, radiotherapeutic, or chemothera-
peutic. Normalization of the prostatic image is seen in
patients sustaining a favorable response to therapy. It is
most likely that changes in the prostate following hormonal
therapy or chemotherapy for metastatic prostate cancer
would mirror the systemic response to therapy, but the
correlation of local and systemic response to treatment
requires further study and analysis.

Finally, there are unresolved problems in the use and
interpretation of transrectal ultrasonography as currently
employed. Most significantly, ultrasonographic criteria
for the diagnosis of prostate cancer are lacking. The
internal echo patterns in particular which characterizes
prostate cancer defy precise definition, and prostate disorders may be identified with high sensitivity but low
specificity. More recent and convincing reports indicate
that most prostate cancers are hypoechoic. Low specificity
also limits the potential use of transrectal ultrasonography as a screening measure. Nonetheless, this imaging
modality holds great promise in the diagnosis, staging,
treatment, and follow-up of prostate cancer.

REFERENCES

Burks DD, Drolshagen LF, Fleischer AC, Liddell HT, McDougal
    WS,Karl EM, James AE,Jr. (1986). Transrectal sonography
    of benign and malignant prostatic lesions. AJR 146:1197-
    1191.
Chodak GW, Wald V, Parmer E, Watanabe H, Ohe H, Saitoh M
    (1986). Comparison of digital examination and transrectal
    ultrasonography for the diagnosis of prostatic cancer.
    J Urol 135:951-954.
Dähnert WF, Hamper UM, Eggleston JC, Walsh PC, Sanders RC
    (1986). Prostatic evaluation by transrectal sonography
    with histopathologic correlation: The echopenic appear-
    ance of early carcinoma[1]. Radiology 158:97-102.
Dähnert WF, Hamper UM, Walsh PC, Eggleston JC, Sanders RC
    (1986). The echogenic focus in prostatic sonograms with
    xeroradiographic and histopathologic correlation.
    Radiology 159:95-100.
Fujino A, Scardino PT (1985). Transrectal ultrasonography
    for prostatic cancer: Its value in staging and monitoring
    the response to radiotherapy and chemotherapy. J Urol
    133:806-810.

Fujino A, Scardino PT (1986). Transrectal ultrasonography for prostatic cancer. 11. The response of the prostate to definitive radiotherapy. Cancer 57:935-940.

Lee F, Gray JM, McLeary RD, Meadows TR, Kumasaka GH, Borleza GS, Straub WH, Lee F,Jr., Solomon MH, McHugh TA, Wolf RM (1985). Transrectal ultrasound in the diagnosis of prostate cancer: Location, echogenicity, histopathology and staging. Prostate 7:117-129.

Lee F, Gray J (1985). Histopathologic-ultrasonographic correlations. Presented at Prostate Cancer Program Planning Meeting. Organ Systems Coordinating Center, Buffalo, NY.

Pontes JE, Eisenkraft S, Watanabe H, Ohe H, Saitoh M and Murphy GP (1985). Preoperative evaluation of localized prostatic carcinoma by transrectal ultrasonography. J Urol 134:289-291.

Resnick MI, Willard JW, Boyce WH (1980). Transrectal ultrasonography in the evaluation of patients with prostatic carcinoma. J Urol 124:482-484.

Spirnak JP, Resnick MI (1984). Transrectal ultrasonography. Urol 23:461-467.

The Use of Transrectal Ultrasound in the Diagnosis and
Management of Prostate Cancer, pages 161-176
© 1987 Alan R. Liss, Inc.

THE UNITED KINGDOM EXPERIENCE : CLINICAL TRIALS FOR
CARCINOMA OF THE PROSTATE MONITORED BY ULTRASOUND

Peeling W B*, Griffiths G J[o], Jones D R[o], Ryan P G*
Roberts E E[+], Evans K T[+]

Departments of *Urology and [o]Radiology, Gwent
Urological Centre, St. Woolos Hospital, Newport,
U.K. NPT 4SZ. [+]Academic Department of Radiology,
University Hospital of Wales, Cardiff, U.K.

In the United Kingdom, many urologists are involved
in clinical trials to test various modalities of treatment
for prostatic cancer. Of these, very few have yet been
able to find the funds for equipment to carry out transrectal ultrasonography of the prostate as a routine process
or within these trials, so that there is little, if any,
accumulated experience to report from Britain in this regard.
However, there has been no lack of interest by British
urologists in transrectal ultrasonography for the limita-
tions of digital palpation of the prostate to obtain
MEASURED DATA about primary prostatic cancer is generally
accepted. Therefore, the advent of transrectal ultrasonography is now regarded as the most promising new method to
obtain the sort of objective information about the size of
the prostate and the internal structure within the gland
that could improve the quality of data entered into clinical trials.

But there are those urologists who question whether
transrectal ultrasonography really offers something in
addition to the traditional clinical method of digital palpation of the prostate to make a diagnosis, to biopsy suspect lesions, and to stage prostatic carcinoma, and to
follow up and assess its response to treatment. In other
words, is the considerable investment in time and money to
set up prostatic ultrasound facilities to monitor patients
with carcinoma of the prostate in clinical trials justified
by a worthwhile improvement in quality of data?

These four aspects will be considered based upon

experience of the Newport/Cardiff group from clinical observations and studies upon cadaver prostates.

Material and Methods
a) Clinical Studies
Between 1978 and mid-1986, 3348 transrectal ultrasonic
scans of the prostate were carried out on 2653 patients.
This series included 221 patients with prostatic cancer with
detailed analysis of acoustic characteristics of their tumours in relation to histological findings. Until mid-1984,
all patients were scanned using a 3.5 MHz chair-mounted probe
coupled to a static scanner using procedures previously described by our group (Brooman et al, 1981). Since 1984, most
patients have been scanned using a 4.0 MHz hand-held probe
(Bruel & Kjaer type 1846). Sixty seven prostatic biopsies
have been carried out under ultrasound guidance since 1985
(by P.G.R) using a modification of the technique described
by Holm & Gammelgaard (1981). Tru-cut needle core biopsies
and fine needle aspiration for cytology were obtained; 51%
of these procedures were performed under local anaesthesia.

b) Cadaver Studies
A pilot study of 10 prostates taken from cadavers reported in 1981 (Brooman et al, 1981) has been followed by a
further study of 100 prostates from cadavers, (Jones et al,
1986). Each specimen was subjected to routine ultrasonic
scanning in a specially designed water tank and in 90 samples histological and microradiographic examination of tissue taken from each level of scanning has been studies. In
this group 26 prostatic cancers were analysed.

RESULTS AND DISCUSSION OF TOPICS
1. Diagnosis and Localisation of Carcinoma of the Prostate
a) Ultrasonic characteristics of prostatic cancer
An analysis of the ultrasonic characteristics of prostatic cancer in the Newport/Cardiff series has recently been
reported by Griffibhs et al (1986). This was based on 221
histologically proven cases of prostatic cancer, of which
96% were hypoechoic 3% were isoechoic and 1% was hyperechoic.
Further analysis in relation to the integrity of the prostatic capsule seen on ultrasound revealed that iso- and hyperechogenicity was only present when the capsule was ultrasonically intact. All patients with capsular discontinuity
on ultrasound, and presumably with locally invasive disease,
had hypoechoic tumours. With regard to localisation of prostatic cancer within the prostate, Griffiths et al (1986)

reported that the ultrasonic abnormalities of many cancers frequently involved more than one quadrant of the prostate, but in tumours confined within the prostatic capsule (Stage T1/T2 : Stage B) ultrasonic abnormalities were more often situated postero-laterally. There was loss of the line of demarcation between periurethral adenomatous tissue and the peripheral zone of the prostate in 70% of patients with cancer and it was considered that this is a valid but not previously reported ultrasonic sign of extensive prostatic cancer.

In the unpublished cadaver prostate study from Cardiff (Jones et al 1986), a similar pattern was evident. Of 26 cases of histologically proven carcinomas of the prostate, 73% were hypoechoic 12% were isoechoic and 15% were hyperechoic. Of these, 13 specimens showed carcinomas with a histologically proven intact prostatic capsule of which 7 (54%) were hypoechoic, 3 (23%) could not be identified ultrasonically and were therefore isoechoic, and 3 (23%) were hyperechoic. The remaining 13 specimens showed discontinuity of the capsular outline on ultrasound, had histological proof of local invasion of the tumour and in 12 of 13 specimens (92%) the echo pattern was hypoechoic. However, 1 specimen (8%) showed hyperechogenicity of the cancer. More detailed examination of hyperechoic lesions by microradiography revealed the presence of microcalcification within these tumours (Fig 1), but histological examination of equivalent tissue in hyperechoic tumours often showed little evidence of microcalcification. This presumably had been excluded from the tissue by the cutting process or washed away in the preparation of the tissue for histological staining.

Microradiography of isoechoic prostatic cancers showed that there was no calcification present in these tumours but that the fine structure of the prostate had been preserved despite the presence of the tumour, and this was similar in texture to surrounding,non-malignant prostate. (Fig 2)

In contrast, tumours that were hypoechoic on ultrasonic scanning, were shown by microradiography to be amorphous in consistency and lacked a fine internal structure within the tumour such as that seen within isoechoic tumours and normal prostatic tissue. (Fig 3)

Discussion
The central issue of concern at the moment is the true acoustic pattern of prostatic cancer. Earlier statements

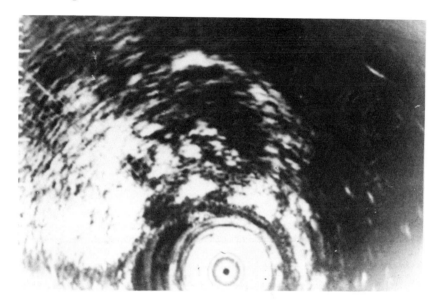

Hyperechoic Ultrasound Scan

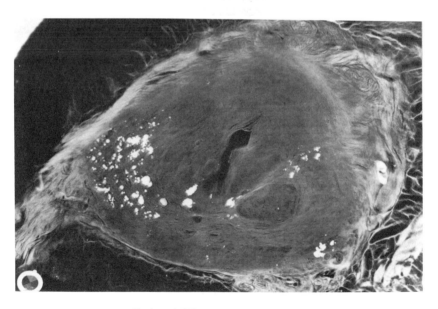

Paired Microradiograph
Fig. 1

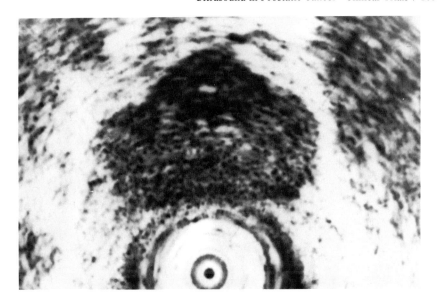

Isoechoic Ultrasound Scan

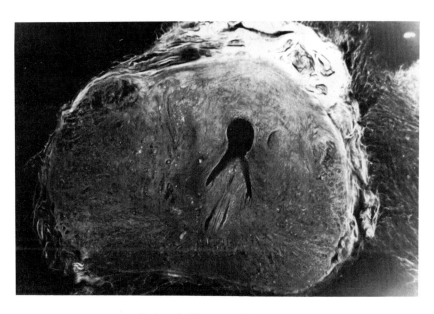

Paired Microradiograph
Fig. 2

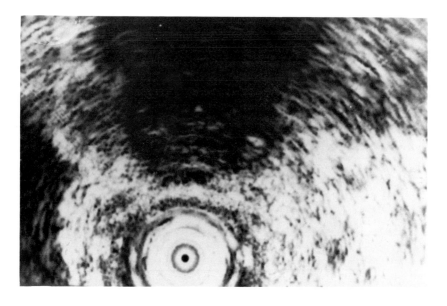

Hypoechoic Ultrasound Scan

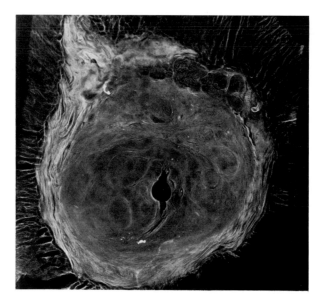

Paired Microradiograph
Fig. 3

maintained that prostatic cancer is hyperechoic relative to
the remainder of the gland (Harada et al 1980, Resnick 1980,
Watanabe et al 1980) or of a heterogenous echo pattern as
described in our previous work (Brooman et al 1981, Peeling
& Griffiths 1984). We therefore agree with Rifkin et al
(1983), Dahnert et al (1986) that most but not all prostatic
cancers are hypoechoic but disagree with Lee et al (1985) in
their statement that all prostatic cancers have hypoechogenic
ultrasound characteristics. In our experience, some isoechoic or hyperechoic tumours occur, and when present have
been cancers confined within the prostatic capsule. Isoechoic lesions occurred in 3% of the clinical series, and
microradiographic studies of similar cadaver speciments revealed that the normal fine structure of the prostate had
been retained within these tumours so that there was no con-
trasting interface that could be revealed by ultrasound.
Hyperechoic lesions were associated with microcalcification
within the tumour and although rare, undoubtedly occur in
clinical practice. These observations might explain the
early interpretation of some cancers as hyperechoic lesions,
or as heterogenous lesions from which positive needle biopsies for cancer had been obtained. It is probable that it
was the echo-poor part of the heterogenous lesions that represented malignant tissue but this was not recognised at
that time.

b) Application of acoustic interpretation to clinical practice
i) Diagnostic Accuracy
   Some reports have presented impressive accuracy rates
for diagnosis of prostatic cancer by ultrasound - 94%
(Watanabe et al 1980), 92% (Resnick et al 1980), 86% (Harada
et al 1980). Such results are impressive, but could digital
palpation have been as good?

   This point was studied some years ago in a study from
our group in which the accuracy of diagnosis of prostatic
cancer when made by digital palpation was compared with the
accuracy achieved by transrectal ultrasonic scanning of the
prostate (Peeling & Griffiths 1984). For 70 men, the respective accuracy rates of diagnosis for prostatic cancer
were 87% for digital palpation against 97% for ultrasound.
Taken at face value, these results would appear to confer
little advantage to ultrasound over digital palpation. However, when the same matter was considered in relation to the
initial diagnosis and staging by the clinician, a different

pattern appeared. It was evident that when the clinician
had made a diagnosis of unconfined, invasive prostatic cancer (T3/T4:Stage C) both digital palpation and ultrasound
had a diagnostic accuracy rate of 96%. However when the
clinician had diagnosed a confined prostatic cancer (T1/T2:
Stage B) by digital palpation, only 50% of these suspected
tumours were ultimately shown by biopsy to have a tumour,
whereas a label of suspected prostatic cancer was correctly
designated by ultrasound to 93% of proven cancers.

Discussion

These observations suggest that transrectal ultrasound
had no part to play in the diagnosis of prostatic cancer
when the tumour was felt to be locally invasive but that it
was most valuable to separate benign conditions from malignant tumours in prostatic lesions considered clinically to
be T1/T2:Stage B cancers.

ii) Biopsy

The indications for ultrasound guided biopsy of the
prostate in our series were (i) the presence of a nodule or
induration on digital palpation of the prostate, or (ii) the
presence of ultrasonic abnormalities suspecting a cancer.
The mean age of 67 patients biopsied was 72 and 51% of these
operations were carried out under local anaesthesia without
undue discomfort or complication. Ultrasound echoes from
fine needles used for aspiration cytology were as clear as
those from larger Tru-cut needles.

Biopsies on 54 patients with a palpable nodule or induration in the prostate were performed using a Tru-cut
needle in addition to fine needle cytological aspiration.
In the Tru-cut needle biopsy group 22 were proved histologically to have prostate cancer whereas from the remaining
32 patients benign tissue only was obtained. With this
technique there were no instances of inadequate tissue cores.
In contrast for these same patients, cytological aspiration
revealed carcinoma in only 13 patients, benign disease in 18,
but from 19 cases the aspiration sample was unsatisfactory
or inadequate for diagnostic purposes. 13 patients were
biopsied for other reasons such as elevated prostatic acid
phosphatase levels, and in none of these was a nodule or induration palpable clinically. In no instance was carcinoma
detected histologically or cytologically by biopsy.

Fifty nine patients in this group were reported to have

ultrasonic abnormalities suspicious of carcinoma for which biopsy was recommended. Carcinoma was proved histologically in 20 patients and a histological report of benign disease was returned in 39. In contrast only 11 patients with carcinoma were detected cytologically in this group, and again there was a high failure rate of sampling for adequate diagnosis. Eight patients had no ultrasonic evidence suspecting carcinoma, and of these 2 were shown histologically to have cancer, and 2 cytological evidence of cancer.

Discussion

In these studies, Tru-cut needle biopsy was more reliable than aspiration cytology in detecting suspected areas of prostatic cancer which were well localised by ultrasound.

2. Staging of Proven Prostatic Cancer

In a patient with proven prostatic cancer, it is perfectly reasonable to regard integrity of the prostatic capsule as demonstrated by transrectal ultrasound to be an indicator of a confined Stage T1/T2:Stage B tumour.

Similarly it is logical to deduce that real discontinuity of the capsular image in association with a proven tumour means locally invasive unconfined cancer (Stage T3/T4: Stage C).

However, there is always the doubt that these images do not represent the real pathological situation within the prostate and firm proof is needed about this.

In Cardiff there has been a major programme to correlate ultrasonic staging with histology in cadaver prostate specimens. Early work reported by Brooman et al (1981) on 6 cadaver prostates containing cancer, has recently been continued by Jones et al (1986) on a further 26 malignant prostates. Therefore 32 specimens with prostatic cancer have been studied. Of 16 specimens with intact prostatic capsules ultrasonically, 11 specimens were staged as Stage B;P2 tumours and 5 were staged as Stage B:P2/3 in which malignant tissue had extended to but had not penetrated through the capsule of the prostate into peri-prostatic fat. Sixteen specimens with discontinuity of the prostatic capsule ultrasonically had histological evidence of tumour penetrating the prostatic capsule and actively invading peri-prostatic fat. They were staged Stage C:P3.

Discussion
        In this study, there was excellent correlation between
ultrasonic staging of prostatic cancer in terms of integrity
of the prostatic capsule, with histopathological staging.

Digital Staging of Prostatic Cancer
        The correlation between digital and ultrasound staging
has been examined by Brooman et al (1981) and Ryan et al
(1986). Although each study differs in minor detail, the
accumulated results involving 139 patients with prostatic
cancer do not change the findings of the individual studies.
Of 139 patients reviewed, a digital staging of locally invasive cancer was made in 72 men. This was confirmed ultrasonically in 54 (75%): however, in the remaining 18 patients
(25%) the prostatic capsule was ultrasonically intact.

        A further 67 patients had been staged digitally to have
confined cancers. Of these 39 (58%) showed intact prostatic
capsules ultrasonically, whereas 28 (42%) showed discontinuity of their capsules on ultrasound.

        There was therefore a disagreement between digital
staging and ultrasonic staging in 46 (33%) of these patients
with the majority difference occurring when the tumour had
been judged on clinical grounds to be confined within the
prostatic capsule.

Discussion
        If it is accepted from cadaver studies that transrectal
ultrasonic scanning of the prostate is a reliable and accurate measurement of tumour stage, then these observations
indicate that digital staging of prostatic cancer is considerably inferior in performance to transrectal ultrasound
scanning for both palpably invasive or confined tumours.

3. Assessment of Response to Treatment
        Declerq & Denis (1978) and Hastak et al (1982) have
demonstrated that transrectal radial scanning of the prostate by serial planimetry is the most accurate method of
measuring volume and volume changes during treatment.

        To examine the accuracy of this process, Jones et al
(1986) in Cardiff measured the volume by ultrasound of 100
cadaver prostates and compared these findings with the actual volume of the gland. Three prostates containing extensive invasive cancers could not be measured by this process

because their margins could not be determined so the total number of specimens examined was 97. There was a close correlation between the physical volume of the prostate and its volume measured and calculated ultrasonically particularly for benign hyperplasia, but the correlation was less reliable for prostatic cancers (Fig 4). Poor correlation was only present in unconfined cancers.

In clinical trials experience with transrectal ultrasonography is limited at the present time to a few centres. We have found it of value in measuring volume in relation to other parameters in trials, as for instance in a recent study of patients treated in phase II and III studies of the effect of the depot formulation of the LH-RH analogue I.C.I.118630 ("Zoladex") and Zoladex against orchidectomy. In these trials 38 patients with metastatic prostatic carcinoma were evaluated. Following treatment there was a consistent mean reduction of the volume of the prostate in association with suppression of plasma testosterone levels to castrate ranges and a fall of plasma prostatic acid phosphatase over a period of 27 months. (Fig 5).

A particular value of transrectal ultrasound could be to compare rates of change of prostatic volume in relation to various modalities of treatment. Our experience suggests that with "Zoladex", volume reduction of the prostate stabilises after about 18 months of treatment. This same trend was demonstrated in a phase III trial of orchidectomy against "Zoladex". As with "Zoladex" there was no further reduction of prostatic volume 18 months after orchidectomy, and the rates of reduction of prostatic volume during the first six months for both treatment modalities were the same.

Carpentier et al (1984) demonstrated with transrectal ultrasonic measurements on 39 patients that rates of change of prostatic volume within six months of starting endocrine treatment could predict prognosis, with greater slopes of the volume reduction curve being associated with longer term survival. Our observations have not supported this interesting work. Thirty one patients treated either by orchidectomy or "Zoladex" showed no significant difference in rates of change of prostatic volume during the first six months of treatment whether the patients' disease progressed within the first twelve months of treatment or remained controlled for longer periods of time.

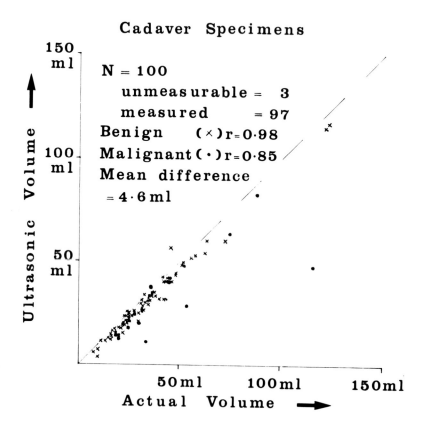

Comparison of Ultrasonic and
Actual Volumes of the Prostate

Cadaver Specimens

N = 100
   unmeasurable = 3
   measured   = 97
Benign   (×)r= 0·98
Malignant(·)r= 0·85
Mean difference
  = 4·6 ml

Correlation between Ultrasound and Physical Volume in
Cadaver Prostates

Fig. 4

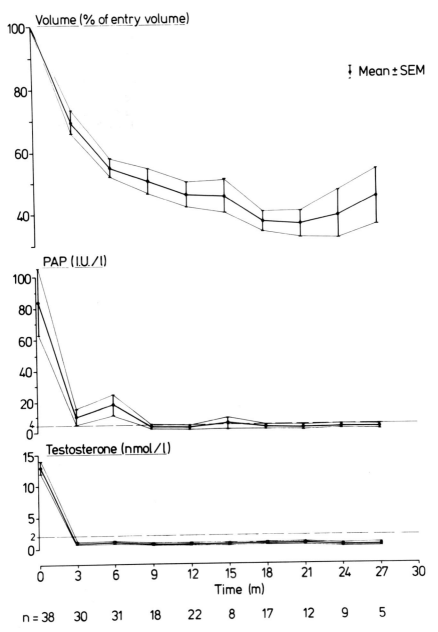

Change in Prostatic Volume, Prostatic Acid Phosphatase, and Testosterone with Time in Treated Prostatic Carcinoma. Fig.5

It might be expected that secondary increase in prostatic volume after a period of suppression of prostatic cancer would predict relapse and escape from control of the disease. This was considered in 50 patients treated with "Zoaldex" or by orchidectomy of whom 17 eventually progressed and died. While these patients were deteriorating, no change in prostatic ultrasonic features occurred in 8 (2 patients consistently had ultrasonically confined tumours), ultrasonic "downstaging" occurred in 7 patients with a change from unconfined to confined features, and only 2 showed an increase in staging from confined to unconfined disease.

Of these patients there were 6 who after a period of treatment had no ultrasonic evidence of malignancy. Of these only 1 had a truly "complete response" to treatment, 4 had active evidence of metastatic disease but were "stable" and 1 progressed to death.

Discussion

These observations support the concept that the behaviour of the primary tumour in prostatic cancer often bears no relationship to metastatic disease. Transrectal ultrasonography scanning of primary prostatic cancer is therefore of no value as an indicator of long term behaviour of prostatic cancer.

The place of transrectal ultrasonography in clinical trials
Conclusion

Experience from South Wales therefore suggests that transrectal ultrasonic scanning of prostatic cancer did not contribute to the diagnosis of Stage C tumours because digital palpation was as effective. Nor was it able to detect sub-clinical cancers on biopsy of apparently normal prostates, and the method did not contribute to the prediction of survival or relapse of patients undergoing endocrine treatment.

On the positive side, transrectal ultrasonography was of undoubted value for the diagnosis of prostatic cancer in those patients with suspect nodules or induration of the prostate, and it was able to localise abnormal areas within the gland for accurate biopsy. Above all else, transrectal ultrasonography was crucial for accurate staging of prostatic cancer. It also has an important part to play in measuring the initial volumetric response to treatment, but only until stabilisation of response had occurred, after which further ultrasonic follow-up scans were of academic interest only and had little practical relevance.

There is therefore a strong case for the use of trans-rectal ultrasound in the INITIAL ASSESSMENT of carcinoma of the prostate, particularly STAGING, in clinical trials. It also has a place for the measurement of initial response of the primary tumour but appears to have little if any useful contribution to make 18 months after treatment has started.

References

Brooman P J C, Griffiths G J, Roberts E, Peeling W B, Evans K T (1981).   Per-rectal ultrasound in the investigation of prostatic disease. Clin Rad 32 : 669-676

Carpentier P J, Schroeder F H (1984). Transrectal ultrason-ography in the follow up of prostatic carcinoma patients: new prognostic parameter? J.Urol 131 : 903-905

Dahnert W F, Hamper U M, Eggleston J C, Walsh P C, Sanders R C (1986). Prostatic evaluation by transrectal sonography with histopathologic correlation : the echopenic appear-ance of early carcinoma. Radiology 158 : 97-102

Declercq G, Denis L (1978). Ultrasonic assessment of pro-static mass. Acta Urol Belg 46 : 74-79

Griffiths G J, Clements R, Jones D R, Roberts E E, Peeling W B, Evans K T (1986). The ultrasonic appearances of prostatic cancer with histological correlation. Clin Rad submitted for publication

Harada K, Tanahashi Y, Igari D, Numata I, Orilasa S (1980) Clinical evaluation of inside echo patterns in gray scale prostatic echography. J.Urol 124 : 216-220

Hastak S M, Gammelgaard J, Holm H H (1982). Transrectal ultrasonic volume determination of the prostate - a pre-operative and post-operative study. J.Urol 127 : 1115-1118

Jones D R, Griffiths G J, Parkinson C, Roberts E E, Evans K T (1986). Unpublished data

Lee F, Gray J M, McLeary R D, Meadows T R, Kumasaka G H, Borlaza G S, Straub W H, Lee F Jr, Solomon M H, McHugh T A, Wolf R M (1985). Transrectal ultrasound in the diagnosis of prostate cancer: location, echogenicity, histopathology and staging. Prostate 7 : 117-129

Peeling W B, Griffiths G J (1984). Imaging of the prostate by ultrasound. J.Urol 132 : 217-224

Resnick M I (1980). Ultrasonic evaluation of the prostate and bladder. Semin Ultrasound 1 : 69-79

Rifkin M D, Kurtz A B, Choi H Y, Goldberg B B (1983).
  Endoscopic ultrasonic evaluation of the prostate using a
  transrectal probe : prospective evaluation and acoustic
  characterisation. Radiology 149 : 265-467
Ryan P G, Griffiths G J, Edwards A, Peeling W B (1986).
  Unpublished data
Watanabe H, Date S, Ohe H, Saitoh M, Tanaka S (1980). A
  survey of 3,000 examinations by transrectal ultrasonotomography. Prostate 1 : 271-278

The Use of Transrectal Ultrasound in the Diagnosis and
Management of Prostate Cancer, pages 177–194
© 1987 Alan R. Liss, Inc.

THE EUROPEAN EXPERIENCE: USE OF TRANSRECTAL ULTRASOUND IN THE DIAGNOSIS AND MANAGEMENT OF PROSTATE CANCER

Dr. med. H. Bertermann

Dept. of Urology

Christian-Albrechts-University, Kiel, Germany

The German History of transrectal prostate scanning (TPS)
began in 1981, when the group of FRENTZEL-BEYME started
their clinical as well as an early detection program
(FRENTZEL-BEYME et al., 1982, 1983). As there have been no
concrete data from the literature on any typical ultrasonic
criteria of prostate cancer except asymmetry of the gland
and capsule penetration, they made a study on autopsy prostates in a waterbath. Using a 3,5 MHz equipment of B & K *,
48 % of small cancerous lesions were hypoechoic, 39 % were
inhomogenous, 13 % were isoechoic compared to the normal
gland, but no hyperechoic cancer tissue could be revealed
(FRENTZEL-BEYME et al., 1982). EGENDER et al. (1983) confirmed the hypoechoisme of prostate cancer in vitro. PEN-
KERT (1983) reported on similar results from ultrasonically
guided perineal biopsies from suspicious echo pattern,
using the technique of HOLM et al. (1981).

From our own experiences with external transvesical scanning of the prostate - without the possibility of guided

*Brüel & Kjaer, Naerum, Danmark

biopsies - we believed that cancer will be hyperechoic
(WENSKY and BERTERMANN, 1982). However, we were convinced
by these first experimentally prooved results from FRENT-
ZEL-BEYME, which were in contrast to the reviewed literature of that time (WATANABE et al., 1975; RESNIK et al.,
1978; HARADA et al., 1980; WATANABE et al., 1980; BROOMAN
et al., 1981).

From transrectal scanning during transurethral resection
of BPH tissue (BERTERMANN et al., 1983) we were forced to
revisualize the data on normal and abnormal growth of the
prostate (Mc NEAL, 1969, 1975; HORIO, 1967): hyperplasia
(BPH) developes in the central inner gland (CG) around the
prostatic urethra between verumontanum and bladder, while
cancer originates from the outer gland, i.e. the peripheral
zone (PZ).

In 1983 and 1984, FRENTZEL-BEYME and BERTERMANN (1) arranged
symposia just on the topic "Prostatasonographie" bringing
together most of the groups of the German speaking countries
working in this field to discuss the controversies. Summing
up, the following "state of art" was acquired: imaging the
prostate, transrectal scanning is much in favour of the
extern transvesical approach, small cancerous lesions are
hypoechoic, bigger tumors often become inhomogenous echo
pattern, computerized post-processing might improve critical
examination, screening for early detection of cancer cannot
be recommended as FRENTZEL-BEYME et al. (1983) could reveal
one nonpalpable cancer from 1024 screened men (with 3,5
MHz), and a stepwise planimetric volumetry is sensitive
against detection of local tumor response or progress

(BERTERMANN et al., 1985). In 1985 we could outline from a waterbath study that hypoechoic lesions within a BPH, which often occur in mixed stromal and glandular hyperplasia, mostly correspond with fibromuscular nodules (BERTERMANN et al., 1985), confirming the results of EGENDER et al. (1983).

THE NATURE OF BENIGN HYPOECHOIC LESIONS

Since 11/85 when we could get a 7 MHz transducer (B & K) with a much more delicate gray scale echo pattern and bringing to mind the normal inner prostatic topography and the origin of alterations such as corpora amylacea and calcifications, smooth muscles round the vesical neck the apical sphincter externus zone and the ejaculatorious ducts, BPH and cancer, we could reduce our rate of false-positive examinations drastically.

Fig. 1 and 2 show the smallest cancerous lesions (5 and 4 mm) provable by ultrasonically guided fine needle biopsies from the perineum.
Fig. 3 shows a central hypoechoic area: this is the urethra with periurethral glands and smooth muscles in a juvenile prostate. Fig. 4 represents small fibromuscular nodules within a hyperplasia of the central gland (BPH), proved by guided transurethral resection.
Fig. 5 reproduces a really black nodule in the dorsal part of the gland, which had been a small abszess (E. colli), successfully treated by local instillation of an aminoglycoside.
Fig. 6. points out hyperechoic and inhomogenous structures in the ventral caudal part of the gland. This has been an Ultrasonic correlate of a focal bacterial prostatitis (trea-

ted by local instillation), fig. 7 shows a tuberculous prostatitis, which looks quite similar to a cancerous lesion.
Fig. 8 demonstrates a small BPH in the ventral part, a bigger cancerous lesion in the left lobe and hyperechoic calcifications in the right lobe (chronical prostatitis).

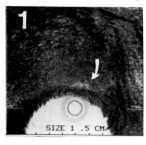

Fig. 1 (7 MHz): Cancer (3x4 mm)
in the left lobe

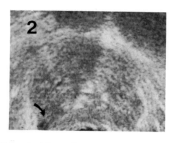

Fig. 2 (7 MHz): Cancer (5 mm) in the
right lobe and BPH (45 ml)

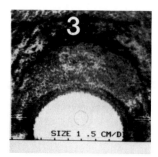

Fig. 3 (7 MHz): Periurethral glands
with smooth muscles: normal hypoechoic area in the central part of the
prostate

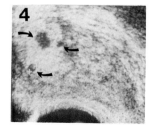

Fig. 4 (7MHz): Fibromuscular nodules
(4-12 mm) within a BPH of 40 ml

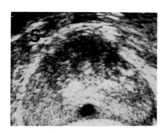

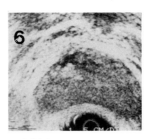

Fig. 5 (7 MHz): Abszess with chronical prostatitis in the central part
(hypoechoic) and diffuse hypoecho-
echogenity (caused by absorption)

Fig. 6 (7MHz): Focal prostatitis
in the ventral caudal area

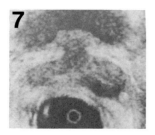

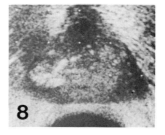

Fig. 7 (7 MHz): Tuberculous prostatitis with hypoechoic areas in the
left lobe of the peripheral zone

Fig. 8 (7 MHz): BPH central and
ventral , cancer in the left
and chronic prostatitis with resulting calcifications in the
right lobe

Our clinical experiences of more than four years with transrectal prostate scanning of more than 1200 patients obvious-
ly reflect the growing developments of ultrasound equip-
ments. For a clinical examination we chequed our TPS-eva-
luations of the last three years.

Tab. I: TPS with 4 and 7 MHz versus palpation in 849 patients with diseases of the prostate

	palpation	transrectal scanning 4 MHz	7 MHz
A: all stages To-4			
n = 214		n = 166	n = 48
false negative	15 %	9 %	4 (2) %
false positive	19 %	11 %	5 %
B: stages To-2			
n = 94		n = 72	n = 22
false negative	38 %	21 %	8 (4) %

From the clinical aspect the advanced stages (t3-4 i.e.
C-D) are of limited interest, because palpation has a sensitivity of nearly 100 %. With 4 MHz we overlooked about
10 % of the palpable cancers, detected on the other hand
every second non-palpable cancer. With 7 MHz, however, we
overlooked only 2 non-palpable cancers: one was an incidental (microscopical small lesion, which is undectable by
ultrasound imaging), the other one was diffusely spread tumor (T2) one year after transurethral resection.

The rate of false positive results is important, too: keep-
ing in mind all the benign origins of suspicious echo pattern, the rate of ultrasonically guided biopsies as well as
the rate of false positive examinations could be kept low.
In case of reasonable doubt a re-examination 1 to 3 months
later will be the adequate decision.

THE BENEFIT OF VOLUME DETERMINATION

The rapid volume estimation following the ellipsoid formula
(latitude x altitude - longitude x 0,523) bears a methodical mistake of 10 - 20 %, increasing in asymmetric organs.
Therefore, we use the <u>stepwise planimetric volumetry</u> (SPV)
consisting of the following procedure (additional need of
time 3 - 5 minutes):
the transrectal equipment is fixed in a stative (fig. 23)
and can be moved stepwise (f.e. 5 mm steps). Beginning at
the apex where just no cross-section of the prostate could
be scanned - this area is called A0 -, all cross-sections
of the prostate were planimetrically plotted by a lightpen
and the volume between the cross-section is automatically
summed up until the final cross-section just beyoned the
vesical neck is plotted (fig. 9 and 10). By the way, all
dots of interest are coordinated three-dimensionally and
could be followed up.
This is the most accepted method of extern volumetry with a
methodical mistake of 5 %.

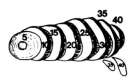

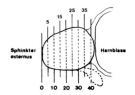

Fig. 9: Schematik drawing of the stepwise
planimetrical volumetry, the stative
is shown in fig. 23.

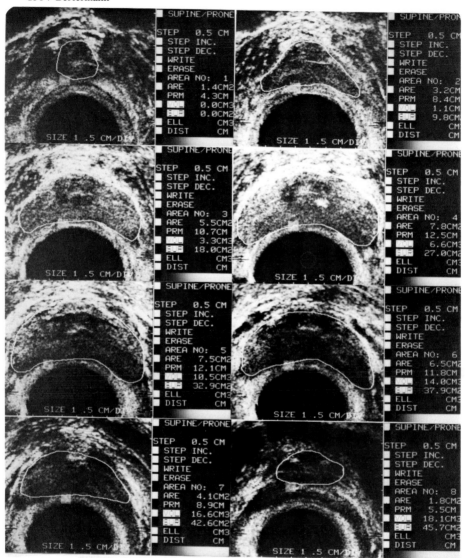

Fig. 10 (7 MHz): Stepwise planimetrical volumetry of a juvenile prostate, final volume: 18,1 ml

Before and during the treatment of prostate cancer we
followed up the volume of the whole gland. Independent of
the kind of treatment (hormonal, radiation), there occured
a rapid and significant decrease of volume within 3 months
when the tumor responded to therapy (fig. 11). Non-respon-
ders led to a constancy and local progression to an increase of volume (fig. 12). Figures 13 - 18 give some examp-
les. It should be emphasized that we could find a nice
correlation with the cytological regression grade (LEISTEN-
SCHNEIDER et al., 1980) and the clinical finding. Beyond
this, a significant increase of volume was the earliest indicator of tumor progression: in 12 cases an average time
of 3 months prior to clinical manifestation.

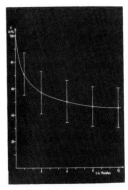 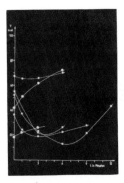

Fig. 11: Volume reduction (in %)
during cancer treatment, plotted
against time of observation (in
months).

Fig. 12: Volume follow-up (in ml)
of cancers with progression, plotted against time of observation
(in months)

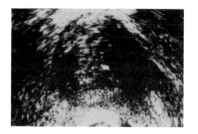

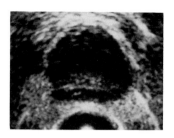

Fig. 13 (3,5 MHz): Cancer in both lobes with infiltration of the left M. obturatorius int., 68 ml

Fig. 14 (4 MHz): Same cross-section after 3 months of treatment, 45 ml

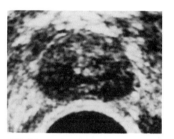

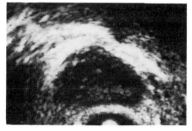

Fig. 15 (4 MHz): Same cross-section after 12 months, 34 ml

Fig. 16 (4 MHz): Same cross-section after 19 months, 23 ml

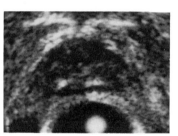

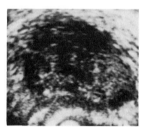

Fig. 17 (4 MHz): Reduced volume (17 ml) after 6 months of treatment

Fig. 18 (4 MHz): Drastical increase of volume (42 ml) after 12 months

Together with a tumor response a normalisation of echopattern could be visualized so that the residual tumor could not further be delineated in most of the cases.
That is the reason why volume studies of the tumor itself failed during the treatment so that an additional fine needle biopsy for a cytological follow up is carried out all 6 months. However, in cases of stable disease with an unchanged reduced volume we dispense with biopsies which tends to increase patients'compliance.

For tumor volume studies in vivo, especially in small cancers, the steps of planimetric volumetry should be 2 mm. We asked already for a modification of the equipment to study the correlation of tumor volume and prostate specific antigen (PSA) levels.

TPS-IMAGES AFTER REMOVAL OF BPH

As an aid for the decision what kind of BPH-removal should be done - transurethral resection (TUR) or an open adenomectomy (PAE) - such an except volume determination as by SPV is not necessary: an extern transvesical ultrasonical volume estimation (ellipsoid formula, s.a.) is sufficient.

But how looks a prostate gland after the PAE of a 95 g specimen? Fig. 19 and 20 demonstrate that 1 month passed the operation the size and shape of the prostate (i.e. the residual peripheral zone) seems to be juvenile: a volume of 25 ml is measured, no bigger cavity is detectable and the reactive increase of volume of the outher gland has disappeared (f.e. total gland: 120 ml, removed adenoma: 95 g, volume of the outher gland 7 days postoperatively: 40 ml).

Quite different is the aspect after a TUR: a comparable reactive increase of the volume of the residual gland could
be observed, but the resection cavity remains wider than
after a PAE and can mostly be demonstrated years after TUR,
especially in the cranial cross-sections (fig. 21 and 22).
This knowledge might be helpfull in avoiding diagnostic
failures.

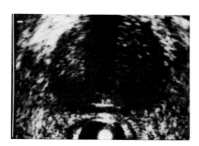

Fig. 19 (4 MHz): Prostate enlarged
by a BPH, 120 ml

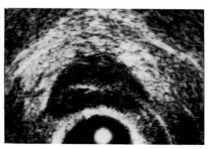

Fig. 20 (4 MHz): Same prostate 1
month after adenomectomy, 25 ml

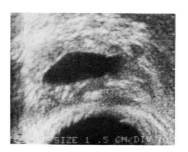

Fig. 21 (7 MHz): Resection cavity
6 month after TUR

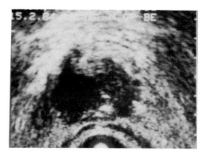

Fig. 22 (4 MHz): Resection cavity
8 month after a TUR: asymmetric because of subtotal resection

PERINEAL AFTERLOADING TREATMENT WITH IRIDIUM[192] IN LOCAL PROSTATIC CANCER

Local disease calls for local treatment.

Inspirations came from the fascinating procedure of HOLM's

perineal seed implantation (HOLM et al., 1983) and the
good results in gynecological tumor radiation by the
afterloading technique. In cooperation with Dr. F. BRIX,
Dr. P. KOHR and Dr. A. QUIRIN from the Department of Radiology in Kiel we started in 8/85 a perineal interstitial
afterloading treatment with Iridium^{192} under transrectal
ultrasonic guidance (BERTERMANN and BRIX, 1986; BERTERMANN
et al., 1986). A similar approach had been reported by
BRAUN et al. (1986).
Following the technique of HOLM we move hollowed needles
of 2,3 mm diameter from the perineum into the prostate. The
exact needle placement is favoured by a modified puncture
matrix (fig. 23 and 24) and is controlled by transrectal
scanning (fig. 26). Then the 10 mCi source of Iridium^{192}
(fig. 25) is automatically driven through the needles into
the tumor and the source remains a predicted amount of time
in the precalculated position following the computerized
doasage calculation. After 4 - 8 minutes this so-called
afterloading radiation treatment is finished and the
needles were removed.

The dosage calculation is based on the stepwise planimetric
volumetry where the surface of the prostate and the spread
of the tumor is plotted. To cover the prostate by this
afterloading brachytherapy with the aimed 15 Gy (1.500 rad),
two to four needles were required. Fig. 27 and 28 repro-
duce such an isodosage calculation. The whole procedure
is repeated two weeks later and is combined with a special
percutaneous radiation technique, the so-called field inte-
grated dosage modification (FIDM) (BRIX et al., 1986).

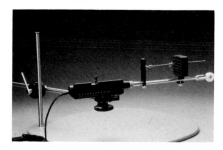

Fig. 23: Stative with stepping unit and puncture matrix

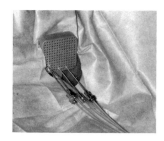

Fig. 24: Modified puncture matrix with hollowed needles, connected with the Iridium^{192} source

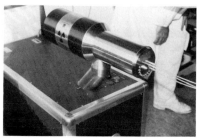

Fig. 25: Iridium^{192} source for afterloading brachytherapy, connected with the needles

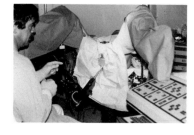

Fig. 26: Patient, equipment and operator in situ

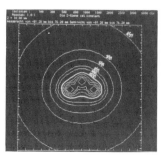

Fig. 27: Cross-sectional isodose simulation with three needles (rhombic symbols)

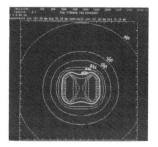

Fig. 28: Plane-sectional isodose simulation of the same case

The indications for such a combined radiation treatment are local tumors (T1-3 No Mo) with an agressive grading (G2-3). The prostate gets 66 Gy (6.600 rad) and the regions of subclinical disease 42 Gy (4.200 rad). In the meantime, 14 patients have been treated in this way. The follow-up is a routinely clinical examination with an additional transrectal volumetry. In all cases a volume reduction of the prostate of more than 20 % within 3 months is observed indicating a local response and no systemical progression could be detected. None of the patient reported any negative side-effects such as local dyscomfort, dysuria, proctitis or any disturbance of sexual function.

As the averagetime of follow-up is only 7 months yet, we cannot serve any definite results. The advantages seem to be that the tumor gets a high radiation dosis, the neighbourhood (bladder and rectum) is not overtreated, asymmetries and infiltrations can be taken into account, the FIDM technique avoids a doasage omission and hyperdosage, no source is left within the patient and the operation staff gets no radiation.

We are hopefull that this procedure will be able to cure even tumors in T3-stages. It might become an alternative for patients who refuse a radical prostatectomy.

References:

BERTERMANN, H., FRENTZEL-BEYME, B. (1983)
"Prostatasonographie", Naerum, B&K-Verlag

BERTERMANN, H., RATHCKE, J., SEPPELT, U., WAND,H. (1983)
Transurethrale Resektion (TUR) eines Prostataadenoms unter
transrektaler Schall-Sicht. In OTTO R CH, JANN Fx (eds.):
"Ultraschalldiagnostik 82", Stuttgart-New York, Thieme,
pp 447-449

BERTERMANN, H., DRAKOPOULOS, A., HOPP, P., DOLZ, N.,
FRENTZEL-BEYME, B., SEPPELT, U. (1985)
Verlaufskontrolle des Prostatakarzinoms durch transrektale
Sonographie. In JUDMAIER (ed.): Ultraschalldiagnostik 84,
Stuttgart-New York, Thieme

BERTERMANN, H., HOPP, P (1985)
Histo- und Sonomorphologie des Prostata-Adenoms. In OTTO
R Ch (ed.): "Ultraschalldiagnostik 85", Stuttgart-New York,
Thieme

BERTERMANN, H., BRIX, F. (1986)
Technik der perinealen interstiellen Iridium[192]-Bestrahlung
des Prostatakarzinoms. Verh Dtsch Ges Urol 38 (in press)

BERTERMANN, H., BRIX, F., KOHR, P. (1986)
Zur kurativen kombinierten Bestrahlung bei lokal begrenzten
Prostatakarzinom. Verh Dtsch Ges Urol 38 (in press)

BRAUN, J., LINDNER, H., KNESCHAUREK, P., SCHÜTZ, W. (1986)
"High-dose-rate" Afterloading-Strahlentherapie des Prostatakarzinoms mit Iridium[192]. Verh Dtsch Ges Urol 37: 535-536

BRIX, F., HEBBINGHAUS, D., JENSEN, J.M. (1986)
Praxisorientierte Hinweise zur Technik der integrierten
Dosismodifikation in einem Teilbereich des Bestrahlungs-
feldes. Strahlentherapie und Onkologie (in press)

BROOMAN, P.J.C., GRIFFITHS, G.J., ROBERTS, E., PEELING,
W.B., EVANS, K. (1981)
Per rectal ultrasound in the investigation of prostatic
disease. Clin Rad 32: 669-676

EGENDER, G., RAPF, C.H., FEICHTINGER, I., MIKUZ, G.,
BARTSCH, G. (1983)
Vergleichende Studien zur Histopathologie und Sonomorphologie der Prostata. In BERTERMANN, H., FRENTZEL-BEYME, B.
(eds.): "Prostatasonographie" Naerum, B&K-Verlag, pp 43-48

FRENTZEL-BEYME, B., SCHWARZ, I., AURICH, B. (1982)
Das Bild des Prostataadenoms und -karzinoms bei der trans-
rektalen Sonographie. Fortschr Röntgenstr 137: 261-268

FRENTZEL-BEYME, B., AURICH, B., DRAUKOPOULOS, A. (1983)
Die transrektale Prostatasonographie in der Krebsfrüher-
kennung. CT-Sonographie 3: 153-158

FRENTZEL-BEYME, B., WEISE, I., REYHER, S., SCHWARZ, J.
(1983)
Zuordnung sonographischer Bilder von Prostata-Erkrankungen
zur Histologie. In OTTO R CH, JANN FX (eds.): "Ultraschalldiagnostik 82", Stuttgart-New York, Thieme, pp 439-442

HARADA, K., TANAHASHI, Y., IGARI, D., NUMATA, I., ORIKASA,
S. (1980)
Clinical evaluation of inside echo patterns in gray scale
prostatic echography. J Urol 124: 216-220

HOLM, H.H., GAMMELGARD, J. (1981)
Ultrasonically guided precise needle placement in the
prostate and seminal resicles. J Urol 125: 385-387

HOLM, H.H., JUUL, N., PEDERSEN, J.F., HANSEN, H., STROYER,
I. (1983)
Transperineal [125]Jodine seed implantation in prostatic
cancer guided by transrectal ultrasound. J Urol 130

HORIO, Y. (1967)
On the morphological alteration of the prostate gland in
aging. Jap J Urol 58: 783-792

LEISTENSCHNEIDER, W., NAGEL, R. (1980)
Zytologisches Regressionsgrading und seine prognostische
Bedeutung beim konservativ behandelten Prostatakarzinom.
Akt Urol 11: 263-271

Mc NEAL, J.E. (1969)
Origin and development of carcinoma in the prostate.
Cancer 23: 24-34

Mc NEAL, J.E. (1975)
Structure and Pathology of the prostate. In GOLAND M (ed.):
"Normal and Abnormal growth of the Prostate". Illinois,
C.C. Thomas, pp 53-65

PENKERT, A. (1983)
Ultraschallgezielte Prostatapunktionen. In BERTERMANN H,
FRENTZEL-BEYME B (eds.): "Prostatasonographie, Naerum,
B&K-Verlag, pp 37-38

RESNIK, M.I., WILLARD, J.W., BOYCE, W.H. (1978)
Ultrasonic evaluation of prostatic nodule. J Urol 120:
86-89

WATANABE, H., IGARI, D., TANAHASHI, Y., HARADA, K., SAITOH,
M. (1975)
Transrectal ultrasonotomography of the prostate. J Urol
114: 734-739

WATANABE, H., DATE, S., OHE, H., SAITOH, M., TANAKA, S.
(1980)
A survey, of 3000 examinations by transrectal ultrasonotomography. The Prostate 1: 271-278

WENSKY, H., BERTERMANN, H. (1982)
Sonographische Befunde bei Erkrankungen von Harnblase und
Blasenhals. Therapiewoche 32: 684-689

The Use of Transrectal Ultrasound in the Diagnosis and
Management of Prostate Cancer, pages 195–208
© 1987 Alan R. Liss, Inc.

THE JAPANESE EXPERIENCE: USE OF TRANSRECTAL
ULTRASOUND IN THE EVALUATION OF TUMOR RESPONSE
TO VARIOUS TREATMENT MODALITIES

Hiroki Watanabe

Department of Urology, Kyoto Prefectural
University of Medicine
Kawaramachi-Hirokoji, Kyoto, Japan 602

SIZE MEASUREMENT OF THE PROSTATE

It is well known that ultrasonic techniques
are able to make precise measurements of the sizes
of various organs. In urology it is of practical
importance to measure the size and weight of the
prostate.

By means of transrectal sonography (TRS),
tomograms can be recorded routinely every 5 mm of
depth of insertion of the transducer into the rectum, on 35 mm black and white film.

The prostatic volume is estimated as follows:
The area of prostatic section on each tomogram
taken at 5 mm intervals is measured by a roller
planimeter. The sum of the area of each section
multiplied by 0.5 can be taken to be the volume of
the prostate. This prostatic volume can be taken
to be approximately equal to the prostatic weight,
because the specific gravity of prostatic tissue
is about 1.0 according to our measurements of
surgically excised specimens[1].

We estimated the diurnal change of prostatic
weight in normal volunteers. The pattern of diurnal change was classified into three types.
They were the so called "Daytime type" in which
the peak was shown at noon, the "Nocturnal type"
in which the peak appeared at midnight, and the

"Unchangeable type" (Fig. 1).

We also estimated the weight of the normal prostate in 348 cases of various ages. The prostatic weight increased rapidly in adolescence and reached a peak at the age of 20. It then decreased gradually and finally at the age of 80 approached a level similar to that for children (Fig. 2)[2].

KINETICS OF PROSTATIC VOLUME IN TREATING PROSTATIC CANCER WITH CASTRATION

The term "kinetics" means a study to investigate a kinetic change of organs or tumors by means of continuous volumetry. As an application of this, we made a study of the kinetics of prostatic volume reduction in treating prostatic cancer[3].

Fig. 3 shows a maximum section of the prostate before and after castration and some months of estrogen administration in a case of advanced prostatic cancer. A marked reduction of the prostatic size is observed.

Sixty-two cases of prostatic cancer in Stages B, C and D, without any prior treatment, were chosen for the investigation. They were treated only by castration, and the volume of the prostate was measured ultrasonically before and after castration very frequently. Measurement was taken almost every day in the first postoperative week and every two days in the second postoperative week. After the third postoperative week it was taken once or twice per week.

Fig. 4 shows the regression curves of the prostatic volume in these cases. It seems that the volume reduced exponentially in each case after therapy, approaching a constant plateau level without exception.

This fact might be analyzed by the following hypothesis: The prostate involved with cancer can be divided into two portions. One is the "effec-

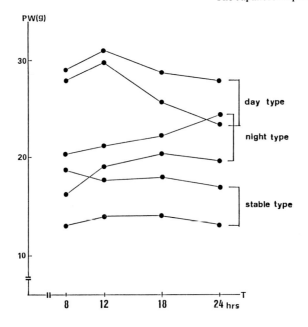

Fig. 1.   Diurnal changes of normal prostatic weight.

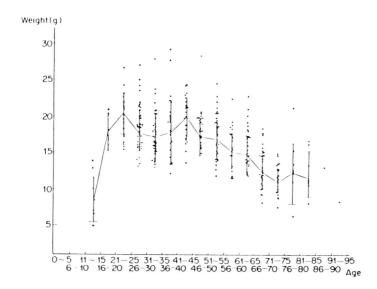

Fig. 2.   Age specific weight of the prostate
          in normal subjects.

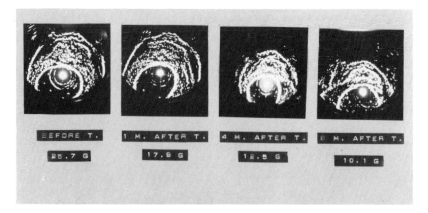

Fig. 3.   Maximum section of the prostate before
and after castration and estrogen administration in a case of advanced prostatic
cancer.

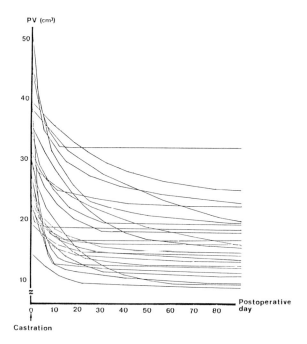

Fig. 4.   Prostatic size reduction after castration
in 24 cases of prostatic cancer.

tive portion" as far as the treatment is concerned, and the other is the "ineffective portion". The volume of the effective portion reduced exponentially to the time elapsed but the volume of the ineffective portion was always constant (Fig. 5).

According to this hypothesis, the regression curves in treating prostatic cancer may have an exponential function which could be expressed as:

$$V = a \cdot 10^{-\frac{t}{\tau}} + b$$

In this formula, "V" is the total volume of the prostate, "a" is the volume of the effective portion, "b" is the volume of the ineffective portion and "τ" is a constant which represents the time interval required for the effective portion to reduce its volume to one-tenth. The dimension of "τ" is [T] and the unit can be expressed by "days". We named this constant the "reduction time" of the effective portion (Fig. 6).

Putting the clinical data of each case into this formula, "τ", "a" and "b" can easily be calculated.

We evaluated the relationship between these three factors; "τ", "a" and "b", and the staging of cancer according to the American classification. Although "a" and "b" showed no remarkable difference between the stages, "τ" in the group of Stage D was nearly double that in the groups of Stages B and C (Table 1). Such a prolonged "τ" means a lower rate of effectiveness of castration.

To confirm the effectiveness of castration in the normal prostate, we calculated these three factors in three castrated beagle dogs using a specially prepared transrectal scanner for the dog prostate[4]. As shown on Fig. 7, "τ" of the dog prostate after castration was rather longer and "b" was remarkably smaller than those in the human prostate with cancer.

In the next step, we evaluated the significance of these three factors for the prognosis of

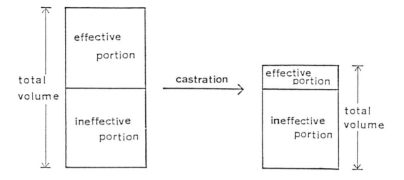

Fig. 5.   Prostatic volume after castration.

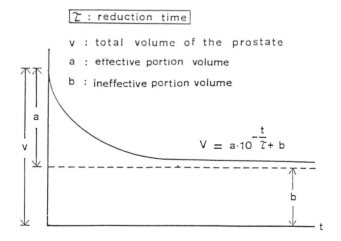

$$V = a \cdot 10^{-\frac{t}{\tau}} + b$$

Fig. 6.   Regression curve of prostatic volume
after castration.

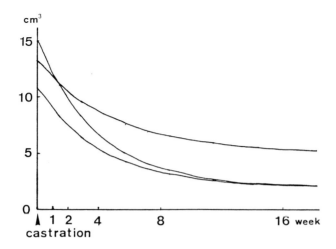

Fig. 7. Regression curve of canine prostate after castration.

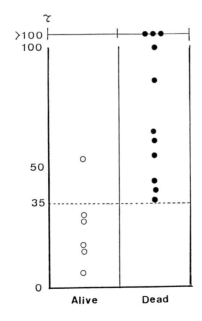

Fig. 8. 7 and 3 years survival in treating prostatic cancer in Stage D.

the patients. Although "a" and "b" were not significant, it was clarified that "ζ" had a very
important role for that purpose. Fig. 8 shows the
relationship between "ζ" and three-year survival
of patients in Stage D. Patients who died of
causes other than cancer were excluded from this
analysis. The "ζ" for the living cases was shorter and that for the deceased cases was longer.
Between them, a clear borderline could be delineated at a "ζ" of 35 days.

Based upon this fact, 5 year survival rates
were calculated according to the acturial method,
in the two groups of patients in Stage D, for whom
"ζ" was over or below 35 days (Fig. 9). A remarkable difference was observed between the two
groups.

At the moment there have been no deaths among
the patients in Stages B and C at the three-year
follow up. Accordingly, an analysis of the significance of the factors in these groups of patients cannot be made for several more years.

In conclusion on the kinetics of prostatic
cancer treated with castration, three points can
be made: first, reduction time, "ζ", which is
calculated from a kinetic analysis of the prostatic volume, is very significant in facilitating a
prognosis of the patient with prostatic cancer.
Secondly, the large majority of patients in Stage
D, having a "ζ" over 35 days, will die within 3
years. And finally, even a patient in Stage D can
survive for more than 3 years, if his "ζ" is below
35 days.

CHANGE OF PROSTATIC VOLUME IN TREATING PROSTATIC
CANCER WITH ESTRAMUSTINE PHOSPHATE

Estramustine phosphate (Estracyt®) is a new
drug which is expected to surpass the conventional
hormonal therapy for prostatic cancer. We evaluated the effectiveness of the drug by means of
ultrasonic measurement.

Forty-four patients with histologically proven prostatic cancer were registered under the cooperation of urological clinics in five medical schools in Japan.[5] They were divided into two groups. One consisted of 37 patients who had received no treatment (study I) and the other of seven patients who had relapsed from prior conventional hormonal therapy with surgical orchiectomy (study II).

Estracyt was administrated orally for over three months in a dose of four capsules (560 mg as estramustine phosphate) a day, or six capsules (840 mg as estramustine phosphate) a day if necessary.

As a rule, TRS was performed before, and one and three months after, the beginning of the treatment. In a limited number of cases, examination was also made six and 12 months after treatment.

As a result, in study I, a remarkable reduction in prostatic volume in each case was found after treatment with estramustine phosphate. This reduction appeared within the first month after the start of treatment. Finally a decrease in prostatic volume could be found in 33 cases (89.2 %) on final examination (Fig. 10).

In study II, a reduction in prostatic volume was noticed in four cases (57.1%). In one of the remaining cases the volume increased, and in the other case it remained unchanged (Fig. 11). The degree of reduction was smaller than in study I.

It must be noted, however, that in study II primary hormonal therapy had been performed and had already had effects on the prostate. The reasonable volume reduction due to conventional therapy, accordingly, might have been accomplished before estramustine phosphate administration. In spite of this, some additional reduction still occurred. It is recommended, accordingly, that this drug might be indicated for use in some cases of prostatic cancer with remission. The indi-

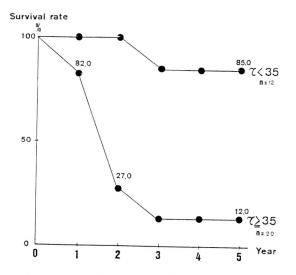

Fig. 9. τ and survival rate in Stage D.

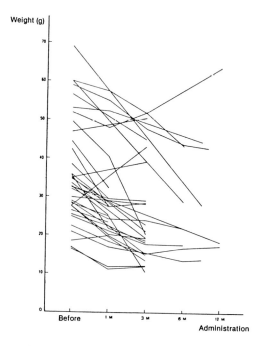

Fig. 10. Change of prostatic weight in study I.

cations can be determined by TRS.

KINETICS OF PROSTATIC VOLUME IN TREATING PROSTATIC
CANCER WITH LHRH ANALOGUE

In a past decade, several derivatives of
luteinizing hormone releasing hormone (LHRH) analogue with high potency have been synthesized and
applied to the treatment of hormone depending disorders including prostatic cancer. Recently,
Ser(Bu)[6]LHRH (buserelin) has been employed in the
treatment of prostatic cancer. We compared a dy-
namic change of prostatic volume with that in serum hormone levels including luteinizing hormone
(LH), follicle stimulating hormone (FSH) and testosterone (T) in the course of the treatment with
buserelin.[6]

Eleven patients with prostatic cancer were
chosen for this study. Buserelin was initially
administered by a subcutaneous injection of 500μg
dose every 8 hours for the first 7 days (n=4) or
14 days (n=7), and then followed by an intranasal
spray of 300μg dose every 8 hours (n=8) or 12
hours (n=3) at least for 4 months.

In all patients examined, continuous daily
administration of buserelin produced relatively
prominent reduction of prostatic volume almost in
parallel with the change of serum T level in the
first month, followed with gradual decline, and
resulted in the minimal value at 4 months later
(Fig. 12).   Decrease of prostatic volume was
62% at the largest and 17% at the smallest (mean
35%) compared with the pretreatment level.

In 5 (Group A) out of 11 cases, the volume of
the prostate increased transiently with a peak on
the 3rd day of the early phase of the treatment,
and then reduced more rapidly than that in the
other 6 cases (Group B) showing no significant
increase of prostatic volume in the same period
(Fig. 13). After the treatment for 4 months, the
prostatic volume of Group A was significantly less
than that of Group B. It may therefore be specu-

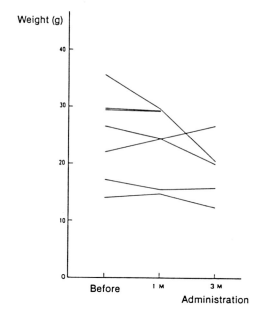

Fig. 11. Change of prostatic weight in study II.

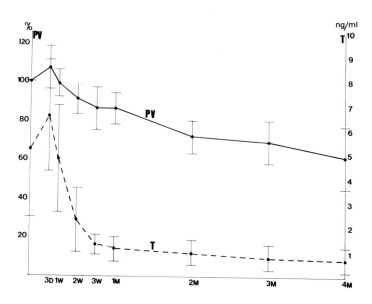

Fig. 12. Prostatic volume and serum testosterone
level during buserelin administration.

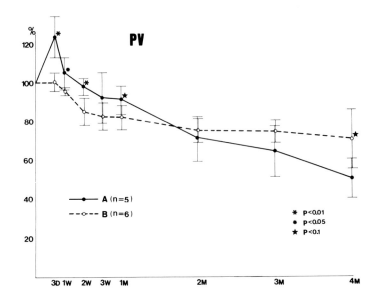

Fig. 13.   Groups A & B in changes of prostatic
volume during buserelin administration.

TABLE 1.   Cases of Prostatic Cancer

Histology / Stage	W.D.	M.D.	P.D.	U.D.	Total
A	0	0	0	0	0
B	7	4	0	0	11
C	10	3	2	0	15
D	8	16	11	1	36
Total	25	23	13	1	62

W.D.: well differentiated
M.D.: moderately differentiated
P.D.: poorly differentiated
U.D.: undifferentiated

lated that prostatic cancer belonging to Group A
is more sensitive to T, and is surmised to result
in better prognosis, than that belonging to Group
B.

A further trial in the future will be needed
to reveal the pathophysiological significance of
kinetic analysis, as done in this study.

REFERENCES

1) Watanabe H, Igari D, Tanahashi Y, Harada K,
   Saitoh M (1974). Measurements of size and
   weight of prostate by means of transrectal
   ultrasonotomography. Tohoku J Exp Med 114:
   277-285.
2) Mori Y (1982). Measurement of the normal prostate size by means of transrectal ultrasonotomography. Jap J Urol 73: 767-781.
3) Ohe H, Watanabe H, Inaba T, Miyashita H,
   Ohnishi K (1985). Relationship between the
   kinetic analysis of prostatic size reduction by
   treatment in patients with prostatic cancer and
   the prognosis. Proc 4th Meeting of the World
   Federation for Ultrasound in Medicine and Biology: p.184.
4) Miyashita H, Watanabe H, Ohe H, Saitoh M,
   Oogama Y, Iijima S (1984). Transrectal ultrasonotomography of the canine prostate.
   Prostate 5: 453-457.
5) Watanabe H, Ohe H, Ando K, Sawamura Y, Niijima
   T, Nakamura S, Orikasa S, Tanahashi Y, Imamura
   K, Yoshida H (1981). The effect of estramustine phosphate on prostatic cancer estimated
   by transrectal ultrasonotomography. Prostate
   2: 155-161.
6) Kojima M, Watanabe H, Ohe H, Miyashite H, Inaba
   T (1986). Kinetic evaluation of reductive effect of LHRH analogue on prostatic cancer using
   transrectal ultrasonotomography. Prostate:
   Submitted for publication.

The Use of Transrectal Ultrasound in the Diagnosis and
Management of Prostate Cancer, pages 209–211
© 1987 Alan R. Liss, Inc.

FUTURE DEVELOPMENTS IN ULTRASONIC IMAGING OF THE PROSTATE

Richard D. McLeary, M.D.

Department of Radiology, St. Joseph Mercy
Hospital, Ann Arbor, MI 48106

Currently available ultrasound equipment is limited by transducers that will image in either the axial or the sagittal plane. Each projection has its advantages and ideally one would like to be able to have both readily available.

The ideal situation would be a biplane transducer capable of obtaining images in both the axial and sagittal planes. This could be done with a variety of schemes, using either mechanical or electronically phased elements.

A prototype biplane device has been developed using 90 degree sector phased array elements. The distal element produces the axial image and the proximal the sagittal. The plane of imaging can be selected from the scanner consol. The main advantage of this device is the ability to image in either projection at will. Each array has a sufficiently rapid frame rate to distinguish blood flow within vessels of the neurovascular bundle as they penetrate the peripheral zone of the gland. This rapid frame rate allows one to conclusively distinguish these blood vessels from other hypoechoic changes within the prostate. (Figures 1-2)

Disadvantages are related to the sector format which requires the transducer to be approximately 2.5cm away from the rectal wall in order to get the entire gland into the field of view in the axial plane.

Steerable range-gated doppler should be able to accurately distinguish vascular structures from solid lesions. It is not out of the realm of possibility that specific doppler signatures may be present that will allow one to differentiate neoplasm from inflammatory or atrophic changes. Doppler may also be able to be used to monitor tumor response to radiotherapy.

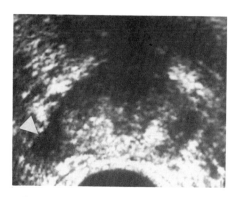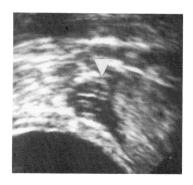

Figures 1,2. Abnormal appearing hypoechoic area on the right side (arrowhead) was noted to be a confluence of blood vessels within which flow could be seen in real time.

One of the tenets of ultrasonic imaging is to use the highest frequency transducer available to image an area of interest. Several whole prostates obtained at radical surgery were imaged at multiple frequencies in a water bath. It appears from this very preliminary work that in the range from 3.5 to 10 Mhz the contrast between neoplasm and normal tissue is inversely related to frequency. (Figures 3-4)

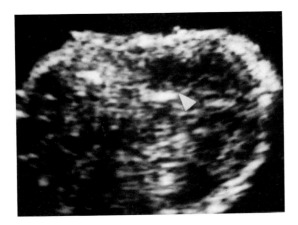

Figure 3. Surgical specimen scanned in a water bath at 5 Mhz. Hypoechoic lesion just to left of midline (arrowhead) is easily seen because of good contrast difference between the tumor and the normal peripheral zone.

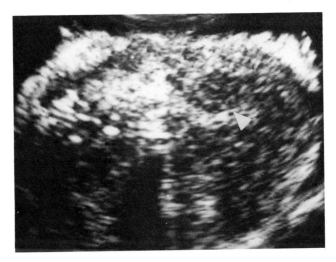

Figure 4. Same specimen as in Figure 3 scanned under the same conditions but with a 10Mhz transducer. The spatial resolution has improved, but the contrast between the tumor (arrowhead) and normal tissue has decreased.

The Use of Transrectal Ultrasound in the Diagnosis and
Management of Prostate Cancer, pages 213–218
© 1987 Alan R. Liss, Inc.

THE DEVELOPMENT OF A THREE DIMENSIONAL PROSTATE MODEL

Peter J. Littrup, M.D.

Department of Radiology, St. Joseph Mercy Hospital,
P.O. Box 995 Ann Arbor, Michigan 48106

Within the last decade, the use of computer aided
graphics in medicine has demonstrated significant clinical
applications. Three dimensional (3-D) anatomic models have
been developed via image reconstruction from various
radiologic modalities (Computer Graphics in Medicine, 1985).
The development of a 3-D prostate model from transrectal
ultrasound (TRUS) data utilizes similar computer graphics
technology. This model has the potential to aid in the
assessment of intraglandular tumor volume and extent.
Appropriate therapeutic options and subsequent follow-up
can then be objectively evaluated.

TRUS evaluation of prostate cancer has indicated
good correlation with histologic size and location on whole
mount studies (Lee et al, 1985). The 3-D model in the
following case presentation was developed in an attempt to
quantify the ability of TRUS to volume prostate tumors.
Further studies are required to define the reliability and
exact correlation of 3-D TRUS analysis and actual tumor
volume.

On routine physical examination, a 59 year old patient
was noted to have a prostate nodule in the left lobe and
referred to a urologist. The nodule was less than 1.5 cm by
palpation and a TRUS examination was ordered for further
evaluation and probable biopsy.

Using a Bruel & Kjaer (B & K) 7 MHz axial transducer,
a suspicious lesion measuring 1.4 cm in width (w) and 1.9 cm
in height (h) was noted in the left peripheral zone (Fig. 1).

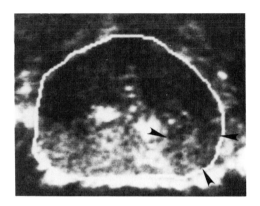

FIGURE 1: Axial scan of the prostate demonstrating a tumor
(arrowheads) in the left peripheral zone.

The tumor margins were not well visualized on sagittal
scanning but a length (l) of 2.5 cm was estimated from
sequential stepping in the axial plane. An average diameter
of 1.9 cm classified this lesion as a ultrasound stage UB2
(Lee et al, Accepted for Publication in Radiology).
Subsequent biopsy revealed well differentiated adenocarcinoma
with a predominate Gleason grade of two and a total grade of
5. A metastatic work-up included a negative bone scan, acid
phosphatase, lymphangiogram, rib films and CT of the pelvis
with contrast.

A TRUS 3-D model was constructed utilizing the voluming
technique on the B & K unit and sequential images were
obtained in 5 mm increments. The central gland, peripheral
zone, and tumor region were outlined for each slice and then
digitized on an Apollo graphics computer* (Fig. 2). A three
dimensional model of the tumor was generated with a calculated
volume of 3.6 cc (Fig. 3). *(Courtesy of the University of
Michigan Architectural Research Laboratory).

Various therapeutic options were discussed and the
patient elected to have a radical prostatectomy. At the
time of operation, pelvic lymphadenectomy revealed no neoplasm
and the prostatectomy was performed without complications. On
pathologic evaluation, the tumor measured 1.5 x 2.7 x 2.5 cm
in greatest dimensions (w x h x l). The height measurement

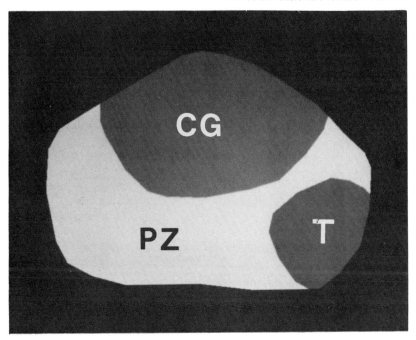

FIGURE 2: Digitized axial image with central gland (CG),
peripheral zone (PZ, and tumor (T) as noted.
Suggested colors: CG - green, PZ - yellow,
T - red.

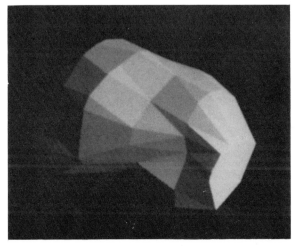

FIGURE 3: 3-D graphic display of TRUS tumor volume = 3.6 cc.

included 0.4 cm of microscopic cellular strands extending anteriorly along the border of the capsule. A 3-D pathologic model was constructed by digitizing the tumor area of each 5 mm tissue section and deriving a total tumor volume of 4.0 cc. The histologic Gleason score was upgraded to a total of 7 and level 3 capsular penetration was noted (Fig. 4). Tumor was found in the margins of resection at the apex of the gland but the seminal vesicles were not involved.

This case demonstrates the prognostic importance of tumor volume with regards to capsular penetration and corroborates recent pathologic studies (McNeal et al, 1986). The 3-D TRUS tumor volume of 3.6 cc approximates the actual histologic volume of 4.0 cc and both models account for the irregular borders of this tumor. The histologic model also included microscopic strands of tumor extension which did not appear to significantly increase the total volume. When the 0.4 cm of microscopic extension is subtracted from the pathologic height measurement, the w, h and l measurements by TRUS show good correlation with the pathologic measurements, ie. 1.4 x 1.9 x 2.5 vs. 1.5 x 2.3 x 2.5, respectively.

The invasive nature of the tumor in this case is supported by the advanced Gleason grade found in the prostatectomy specimen. The lower Gleason score on the initial biopsy probably represents a sampling error within the tumor. The principle of dedifferentiation with tumor growth has been described (McNeal, 1969; McNeal et al, 1986) and a higher tumor grade perhaps could have been expected with a 3-D TRUS volume of 3.6 cc. A cubic volume of 6.7 cc could have been obtained from the product of the TRUS measurements (1.4 x 1.9 x 2.5), but this volume may over-estimate any potential local extension and/or lymph node metastases. For localized tumors of the prostate, the use of TRUS 3-D voluming techniques may thus provide the best estimate of potential histologic invasiveness.

TRUS derived tumor volumes could thereby aid in the selection of patients for either radical prostatectomy or interstitial radiation therapy. The patient in this case demonstrated histologic stage C disease according to the Whitmore staging system (Whitmore, 1956), and will receive a course of external beam irradiation to cover any occult local extension or lymph node metastases. By reserving

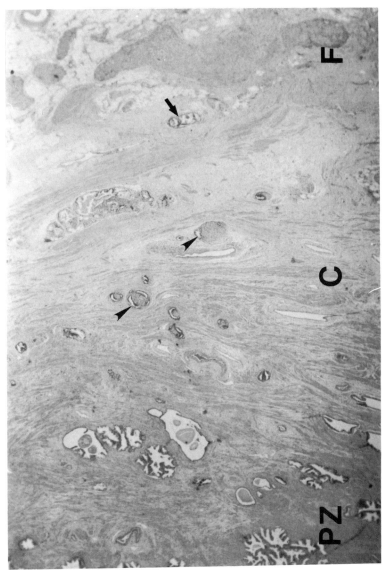

FIGURE 4: Photomicrograph illustrating level 3 capsular penetration. Peripheral zone (PZ), fibromuscular capsule (C), periprostatic fat (F), perineural tumor invasion (arrowheads), tumor in periprostatic fat (arrow).

radical prostatectomy for patients with tumor volumes less than 3.0 cc (stage UA and UB1), the curative potential of this procedure may be increased.

In radiation therapy, a TRUS 3-D prostate model will be very useful in the planning of I-125 seed implantations. Localized interstitial therapy can be devised so that the isodose curve of the I-125 seeds will cover the tumor region accordingly. A follow-up TRUS examination after local edema has resolved could determine if any shifting of the seeds produced "cold" spots in the tumor. Localization data correlation can also be performed by obtaining a CT of the pelvis at 3 mm slices to assess seed location. The resultant isodose model can then be superimposed onto the 3-D TRUS model to further assess adequate coverage. Additional seeds may be placed under ultrasound guidance into any apparent areas of inadequate dosing. In this manner, localized tumors of the prostate will receive definitive irradiation, which may lower the local tumor recurrence rate for interstitial therapy.

REFERENCES

Computer Graphics in Medicine (December, 1985). IEEE CG & A, pp 11-57.

Lee F, Gray JM, McLeary RD, Meadows TR, Kumasaka GH, Borlaza GS, Straub WH, Lee F Jr, Solomon MH, McHugh TA, Wolf RM (1985). Transrectal ultrasound in the diagnosis of prostate cancer: Location, echogenicity, histopathology and staging. Prostate 7:117-129.

Lee F, Littrup PJ, McLeary RD, Kumasaka GH, Borlaza GS, McHugh TA, Soiderer MH, Roi LD (1986). Needle aspiration and core biopsy of prostate cancer: Comparative evaluation using biplane transrectal ultrasound guidance. Accepted for publication by Radiology.

McNeal JE (1969). Origin and development of carcinoma of the prostate. Cancer 23:24-34.

McNeal JE, Kindrachuk RA, Freiha FS, Bostwick DG, Redwine EA, Stamey TA (1986). Patterns of progression in prostate cancer. The Lancet 11:60-63.

Whitmore WF (1956). Symposium on hormones and cancer therapy, "Hormone therapy in prostate cancer". Amer J Med 21:697.

The Use of Transrectal Ultrasound in the Diagnosis and
Management of Prostate Cancer, pages 219–221
© 1987 Alan R. Liss, Inc.

CONFERENCE SUMMARY

Gerald P. Murphy, M.D., D.Sc.

State University of New York at Buffalo,
School of Medicine, Buffalo, New York 14214

The summary of this Conference might well be approached from a number of different directions. Without question
we have had the privilege of specific presentations contained in this book from ongoing work in the United States
from our European and Japanese colleagues, both addressing
the principles of ultrasound, either transaxially or sagit-
ally and other important issues such as the technique of
biopsy and aspiration techniques. We have heard, and undoubtedly will hear more, about the importance of intraprostatic lesions, their visualization by various techniques and their confirmation histologically by various
means. However, despite all this great progress and
despite the many contributions at the present time we have
rather minimal data. We have admittedly collectively had
a very short follow-up. It is appropriate, nevertheless,
to plan for the future to continue to design trials,
clinical investigations, and the care of groups of patients
as well as individuals with this modality in mind. By no
means to my impression is anyone specifically in a public
health sense proposing this modality at the present time
as an easy and simple replacement for any of the existing
diagnostic techniques, be they digital examination, radiographic or radioisotopic, or even the various markers e.g.,
PA or PAP from various blood tests. Rather, various
endeavors have been attempted and various other approaches
are underway. With the improvement of technology and the
equipment available there is no question that this particular conference will mark a start for future contributions.
It is impossible to demand or even request standardization
of techniques for utilization of common staging phenomena by

ultrasound unless future data and additional material are
shared and prospectively planned. This conference will
contribute a great deal to those who wish to proceed on
the basis of this information. However, there are many
centers and individuals throughout the United States who
are already engaged in the application and testing of how
far ultrasound can go to a possible confirmation of pre-
clinical staging, following the response to treatment in
terms of the primary therapy, and following in response to
primary therapy such as radiation treatment, or, for that
matter, detection of local recurrence following surgery
or other techniques. These results are reported herein,
as they are now available.

Perhaps the potential bone of contention really deals
with so-called screening for prostate cancer, a term which
has both public health and research and clinical investigation connotations. It cannot and should not be used
lightly. In the opinion of some this would mean the
distinction of those people or identification of those
groups of individuals who are either symptomatic or asymp-
matic. To my own mind this must involve consideration in
the future of a multi-center trial utilizing the best
equipment available with common internal standards of
individuals who are between 40 or 50 years of age
and without known prostatic diseases. These should include
individuals without a history or knowledge currently of
benign prostatic hypertrophy or prostatitis. They should
be a group of individuals, of course, including black
American males who have the highest incidence of prostate
cancer in the world. Thus, from several centers a group of
asymptomatic, heterogenus Americans, both high risk and
low risk, should be included as part of their regular
physical exam in some sort of serial evaluation for
several years. This of course is clinical investigation.
It is not an answer to a question nor the solution of a
problem. It is, however, hopefully an orderly way to
proceed. One feels confident that that potential might be
realized based upon the contribution of this conference.
We are deeply indebted to Professor Watanabe and our
European colleagues for their contributions already made
in this field. Unfortunately all could not be represented
at this Conference, nor necessarily their specific contributions included. Nevertheless they are a vocal and key

point. Hopefully and collectively we will proceed to
examine this new technology. The examination should include
the applications both in the clinic by radiologists,
urologists and all of us interested in the health of the
American male. Faced with this most important cancer and
with the declining incidence of lung cancer the potential
for extended longevity is such that we deal with this
serious issue. Prevention is desirable but one does not
know how to proceed specifically in this particular case.
Earlier detection has always been one way that has been
sought. The proof of course that it will be beneficial
comes only again by specific multicenter trial. I hope
from this conference such preparations indeed will be made.
One is very optimistic that this might be the case.

Index